"If you're one of the millions afflicted with fibromyalgia or chronic fatigue syndrome, or think you may be, start changing your life for the better now by reading this crucial book. There are very real answers that will help you even more than you dare to hope, and Mary Shomon has done an absolutely masterful job of providing them to you here."

—Dr. Joseph Mercola, author of the *New York Times* bestselling *The No-Grain Diet*

"In line with her other well-researched and empowering books, Mary Shomon's *Living Well with Chronic Fatigue Syndrome and Fibromyalgia* addresses subtle underlying health issues that modern medicine misses. At last, an extraordinary—yet down-to-earth—approach to some of our most complex and frustrating illness."

—Richard Shames, M.D., and Karilee Shames, R.N., Ph.D., authors of *Thyroid Power*

"I can think of few conditions more challenging to patients and the medical profession than fibromyalgia and chronic fatigue syndrome. Once again Mary Shomon has shed an incredible light on what really matters—everything from how to get an accurate diagnosis to finding the best treatment."

—Marie Savard, M.D., author of *How to Save Your Own Life*

"Mary Shomon has done the homework for chronic fatigue syndrome and fibromyalgia patients, talking to hundreds of experts, reviewing thousands of resources, and putting it all together in this easy-to-follow guide. Patients can quickly assess the many conventional and alternative diagnosis and treatment options for these complex, difficult-to-diagnose conditions, saving their time and energy for getting well."

—Stephen E. Langer, M.D., author of *Solved: The Riddle of Illness*

"Fibromyalgia and chronic fatigue syndrome confuse many doctors, and in turn they have difficulty giving good explanations to patients. Mary Shomon has been able to convert this 'medicalese' into simple talk that all patients can understand."

—Kenneth N. Woliner, M.D.

"*Living Well with Chronic Fatigue Syndrome and Fibromyalgia* is a must-read not only for those suffering from CFS and fibromyalgia but also for those practitioners who treat these illnesses. This book provides a road map and gives hope to those struggling with chronic illness."

—David Brownstein, M.D., author of *The Miracle of Natural Hormones*

"Mary Shomon has done it again! She has provided a unique, well-written, and user-friendly guide to the diagnosis and treatment of chronic fatigue syndrome and fibromyalgia, conditions that are generally ignored or mismanaged by conventional medicine. With a wealth of the latest scientific information and a wonderful personal touch, she empowers you to take control of your conditions. At the time when you need it most, she introduces you to FMS and CFS, helps you get diagnosed, and then provides you with all the tools you need to carefully craft your own comprehensive wellness and healing plan and confidently carry it out with the aide of your practitioners."

—Hyla Cass, M.D., author of *Natural Highs*

LIVING WELL WITH
Chronic Fatigue Syndrome and Fibromyalgia

Also by Mary J. Shomon
Living Well with Hypothyroidism
Living Well with Autoimmune Disease

LIVING WELL WITH
Chronic Fatigue Syndrome
and Fibromyalgia

What Your Doctor

Doesn't Tell You . . .

That You Need to Know

MARY J. SHOMON

Quill

A HarperResource Book

An Imprint of HarperCollins*Publishers*

HarperCollins books may be purchased for educational, business, or sales promotional use. For information, please write: Special Markets Department, HarperCollins Publishers Inc., 10 East 53rd Street, New York, NY 10022.

FIRST EDITION

Designed by Joy O'Meara Battista

Printed on acid-free paper

Library of Congress Cataloging-in-Publication Data

Shomon, Mary J.
    Living well with chronic fatigue syndrome and fibromyalgia : what your doctor doesn't tell you . . . that you need to know / Mary J. Shomon.
        p.   cm.
    Includes bibliographical references and index.
    ISBN 0-06-052125-2
    1. Chronic fatigue syndrome—Popular works.   2. Fibromyalgia—Popular works.   I. Title.

RB150.F37S56   2004
616'.0478—dc22

                                                              2003056653

04   05   06   07   08   WBC/RRD   10   9   8   7   6   5   4   3   2   1

For Jon and Ric,
the gentlest of men,
and two calm, loving, and truly healing forces
in my life and in this world

CONTENTS

ACKNOWLEDGMENTS

This book would not have been possible if not for the vision and talent of my editor, Sarah Durand, and the friendship, support, and hard work of my agent, Carol Mann. Special thanks to both for their patience and understanding as I finished this book after the death of my mother.

An extra-special thank-you to my family, Jon and Julia Mathis, who very graciously supported me and gave me the precious time to work on this book. Yes, Julia, Mommy probably *does* work more time than most people!

Love and thanks go to my dear aunt, Rita Kelleher, who always tells me that it's in my genes to write, and who turns a mean phrase herself! I'm so grateful to have Jeannie Yamine, my dearest friend and sister in my life—she is my rock and Richelieu. Thanks to my father and brother, Dan Shomon, Sr., and Dan Shomon, Jr., for their faith and support. And thanks to my in-laws, Barbara and Rus Mathis, who provided a comfy and welcome getaway for my husband and daughter during several of my work-bound weekends.

And more than ever, for my mother, who always believed in my work and mission. I know that she's with me now in spirit, and still giving me "smarts."

Many thanks to Rosario Quintanilla and Elizabeth Mensah-Engmann, who helped keep my daughter safe, entertained, and well cared for while "Mommy made another book!"

Thanks to trainer extraordinaire Silvia Treves, who has kept my joints and body healthier and my spirit brighter, and who has taught me the joy of strengthening my "powerhouse." Dr. Bob Umlauf helped me get and stay focused with his sensible and calming advice. And thanks to Kate Lemmerman, M.D., Scott Kwiatkowski, D.O., and Angela Cannon, who do such a brilliant job of helping me to live well.

A particular thanks to writer, patient advocate, and my friend, Lisa Lorden, who provided a great deal of valuable research and input for the book. (I couldn't have done this without you, Lisa!)

Several people never fail to inspire me. Jacob Teitelbaum, M.D., has shared his great compassion for chronic fatigue syndrome and fibromyalgia patients, and his immense wisdom and intuitive sense regarding diagnosis and treatment. Ric and Diane Blake are so courageous, warm, witty, and vital in so many ways as they go about changing the world. And my friends Gen Piturro and Demo DeMartile are passionately changing the world for the better, both inside and out, and helping so many on the way.

For Laura Hillenbrand, an inspiring and insightful author, who graciously spent some of her precious energy to share her thoughts with me and her fellow CFS patients. We are all so inspired by her strength, wisdom, accomplishments, and eloquent writing.

I also want to thank writer Alice Lesch Kelly and the National Fibromyalgia Association's Lynne Matellana for information, time, and support.

Many thanks to the talented healers and practitioners who so willingly and generously shared time and information: Gina Honeyman-Lowe, John Lowe, Sibyl McClendon, Joseph Mercola, Rich Fogoros, David Brownstein, Mike McNett, Ken Woliner, Viana Muller, Marie Savard, Richard and Karilee Shames, Hyla Cass, and Ann Louise Gittleman.

Thanks also to the many friends and colleagues who helped with research, technical support, friendship, encouragement, and inspiration, including Kim Conley, Kim Carmichael Cox, Laura Horton, Jane Frank, Jody LaFerriere, Vickie Queen, Jim Scheer, Sharon Stenstrom, Ann Welch, Julia Schopick, and my online community of girlfriends, "The Momfriends."

And for the millions of people who live with chronic fatigue syndrome and fibromyalgia, and the hundreds who gave their time and precious energy to share their stories with me for this book, I send my thanks, and my fervent wish that you find the answers you seek and the wellness you so deserve as soon as possible.

FOREWORD

Chronic fatigue syndrome and fibromyalgia unnecessarily cripple an estimated 6 to 12 million Americans. Characterized by exhaustion, "brain fog," insomnia, and—in those with fibromyalgia—widespread pain, these illnesses have been poorly understood by both the medical profession and patients. This has resulted in much unnecessary frustration and suffering.

It is important to recognize that these syndromes can be caused and aggravated by a large number of different triggers. This makes evaluation and treatment more complex in chronic fatigue syndrome/fibromyalgia than in most other illnesses. But a new day is dawning for chronic fatigue syndrome and fibromyalgia treatment. When all the different contributing factors are looked for and treated effectively, patients improve significantly and often get well. Fortunately, Mary Shomon's book will dramatically simplify this process for you.

My experience in treating thousands of patients has shown that chronic fatigue syndrome and fibromyalgia are a mix of many different processes that can be triggered by many causes. Some of you had your illness caused by any of a number of infections. In this situation, you can often define the time that your illness began almost to the day. This is also the case in those of you who had an injury—sometimes very mild—that was enough to disrupt your sleep and trigger this process. In others, the illness had a more gradual onset.

This may have been associated with hormonal deficiencies (e.g., low thyroid, estrogen, testosterone, cortisone, etc.) despite normal blood tests. In others, it may be associated with chronic stress, antibiotic use with secondary yeast overgrowth, and/or nutritional deficiencies. Indeed, we have found well over fifty common causes of, and factors that contribute to, these syndromes.

What these processes have in common is that most of them can suppress a major control center in your brain called the hypothalamus. The center is similar to a fuse box in your house. When your body is subject to too much stress (physical or situational), it can "blow a fuse." Your hypothalamic "circuit breaker" controls sleep, your hormonal system, temperature, and blood flow/blood pressure. When you don't sleep deeply, your immune system also stops working properly and you'll be in pain. Although devastating (all the lights go out), having a circuit breaker go off protects the wiring in the house. In the same way, developing chronic fatigue syndrome and fibromyalgia can actually protect your body from further harm. This does not help you, however, unless you learn how to turn the circuit breaker back on. Basically, my approach to doing so rests on four key elements: (1) establishing restorative sleep quality and quantity, (2) correcting hormonal imbalances, (3) eliminating viral, bacterial, and parasitic infections, and (4) correcting nutritional deficiencies and imbalances with appropriate supplementation.

My research team and I have had the privilege to conduct a scientific study of this approach, and the resulting research project is profiled in this book. Our findings were featured as lead article in the *Journal of Chronic Fatigue Syndrome*. The article, titled "Effective Treatment of Chronic Fatigue Syndrome and Fibromyalgia—the Results of a Randomized, Double-Blind, Placebo-Controlled Study," showed that over 90 percent of patients improved with a multidisciplinary treatment approach, and with two years of treatment, the average improvement in quality of life was 90 percent, with a 50 percent reduction in pain, on average.

That the vast majority of patients in my study improved significantly in the active group while there was minimal improvement in the placebo group proves two very important things. The first is that these are treatable diseases. The second is that anyone who now says that these illnesses are not real or are all in your head are clearly both wrong and unscientific.

In addition to my successful multidisciplinary approach, there are many other treatments available as well, and this book does a superb job of reviewing them! It would literally take you thousands of hours to do the research that went into making this book.

I have known hundreds of researchers and workers in this area. Sadly, much of what people write about is directed by politics, institutional dogma, money, and sometimes just plain, old-fashioned closed-mindedness. It has been very refreshing to get to know Mary Shomon. She is an intensely committed woman whose work has simply been guided by love, truth, and compassionate caring. She brings a sharp mind and an open-minded skepticism to the chronic fatigue syndrome/fibromyalgia literature and community and manages to pull all this off with incredible grace! Mary Shomon's work is very balanced, with her only bias being what works, and what is safe and worthwhile. Because of this, you can now get well without having to go out and get your own M.D. or Ph.D.!

At this time, you have all the tools you need to get well now! We wish you all God's blessings and our best wishes in reclaiming vibrant health!

With appreciation for all you've been through,

—Jacob E. Teitelbaum, M.D.

Dr. Jacob Teitelbaum is a board-certified internist and director of the Annapolis Research Center for Effective CFS/Fibromyalgia Therapies. After suffering with and overcoming these illnesses in 1975, he has spent the last three decades creating, researching, and teaching about effective therapies. His clinic is in Annapolis, Maryland. He lectures internationally, and is the author of the best-selling book *From Fatigued to Fantastic!* and his newest book *Three Steps to Happiness—Healing through Joy!* focuses on how to get a life you love. He has also formulated two products specifically for chronic fatigue syndrome and fibromyalgia: "Revitalizing Sleep Formula," and "The Energy Revitalization System" vitamins, both by Enzymatic Therapy, with 100 percent of the royalties from his products going to charity. His Web site is located at www.vitality101.com.

In the fell clutch of circumstance
I have not winced nor cried aloud.
Under the bludgeonings of chance
My head is bloody, but unbowed.
. . . .

It matters not how strait the gate,
How charged with punishments the scroll,
I am the master of my fate:
I am the captain of my soul.

—WILLIAM ERNEST HENLEY, *Invictus*

1

Introduction

Better than a thousand useless words
is one single word that gives peace.
—The Dhammapada

As I started the process of writing this book, I was confused and overwhelmed. For several years, I had been studying everything I could find about chronic fatigue syndrome (CFS) and fibromyalgia. I read more than fifty health and medical books, a thousand medical journals and magazine articles, and two thousand personal e-mails from people with CFS and fibromyalgia. I heard from dozens of experts from around the country. And as I sat down to write, I struggled with a fundamental challenge: All the books, articles, experts, and patients rarely agree on the answers to even the most basic questions.

What are the symptoms of CFS or fibromyalgia? Are CFS and fibromyalgia actually the same disease? How do you get diagnosed? Why would some doctors suggest that CFS and fibromyalgia are just "fad" illnesses, and all in your head? Do you need blood tests or not? What are some of the triggers? Is it stress? Nutritional deficiency? Toxic exposure? Infection? Can you ever get better? What treatments are best? Should you follow a holistic, natural, or alternative medicine approach?

Or forget holistic, should you go totally conventional and take prescription antidepressants, prescription sleeping pills, and prescription pain relievers? Is it all really about an underlying endocrine or thyroid imbalance, and are hormones the answer? Is the solution the guaifenisin protocol, or is it detoxification? Is exercise helpful or harmful? What about your diet and vitamins? Could psychotherapy be the solution? Could you be dealing with a virus, a bacterial infection, a stealth pathogen? Should you have surgery or is the real answer yoga, cranial manipulation, or trigger point therapy?

One patient, BJ, struggled to get a doctor to take her seriously.

I find doctors simply are not interested in this illness. There are no dramatic treatments so there can be no heroes.

While there may not be any heroes, there are some experts who are standing out, taking risks and offering more than just the standard fare, when it comes to CFS/fibromyalgia treatment. But whom should you believe? Should you listen to Dr. Teitelbaum, or Dr. Cheney, or Dr. St. Amand, or Dr. Lowe, or Dr. Bell, or any one of the other CFS and fibromyalgia experts? Should you listen to your own G.P., or your rheumatologist, or your internist, or your infectious disease specialist, or your chiropractor, or your holistic M.D.? Will you be able to find a doctor who cares about *you*?

Just trying to sort through this all gave me a huge headache. (Headache, by the way, can be a symptom of CFS and fibromyalgia, depending on which expert you consult!) But in my case, headache was a symptom of *information overload and confusion*.

I know that you can relate to what I'm saying. For those of you who are in the throes of CFS or fibromyalgia right now—whether you're struggling to get a diagnosis, you've just been diagnosed, or you're a long-term traveler on the road to better health—a headache is the least of your problems. Not only are you suffering a variety of symptoms, which may include total and utter fatigue and exhaustion, difficulty or impossibility concentrating, and debilitating pain, among others, but on top of it all, if you're going to feel better, you have to take charge of your own health and learn all about CFS or fibromyalgia yourself! And all this while you struggle with conditions that, despite their very real and demonstrable existence, carry an outdated stigma not seen with other conditions. With CFS and fibromyalgia, there will always be doctors, family members, and friends who dismiss you as lazy or suffering from a psychosomatic illness, or who assume that if you'd just pull yourself together, you'd feel better.

You probably feel confused, as I was, by all the conflicting information, and overwhelmed by all the options you have and choices you have to make. And more than most conditions, CFS and fibromyalgia require an educated, involved, and empowered patient.

The hardest part is that you need to tackle this huge challenge at a time when you're most likely feeling sick, exhausted, fuzzy-brained, and in pain.

Talk about a *wrong* time to try to delve into a complicated medical topic! Learning about and tackling chronic illness may seem like more than you can handle, especially when it may be overwhelming to think about performing even the most basic activity, such as getting out of bed or brushing your teeth.

You may also be surprised at what a stigma CFS and fibromyalgia still have. You're going through it, so you know from firsthand experience that these are very, very real conditions. You didn't dream this up, wish it upon yourself, or develop some psychosomatic syndrome, and you can't just think it away, buck up and feel better, or "get over it" by sheer determination.

Many people—including some doctors—still think that chronic

fatigue syndrome is the yuppie disease, and that somehow you bring it upon yourself. The problem is, people who think you bring it upon yourself also seem to think that you can easily will it away.

Others think that rather than real, diagnosable diseases, CFS and fibromyalgia are actually psychosomatic and due to laziness, malingering, or some inherent emotional or character weakness.

This is amazingly discouraging when it's coming from friends, family, and coworkers, much less your doctors and practitioners.

It's hard for some people to believe you are sick, and this is one of the most discouraging aspects of CFS and fibromyalgia. You probably appear well, even if you are quite ill and unable to function. The fact that these conditions are not visible contributes to the lack of respect you may experience from others.

Jessica, a CFS patient, said:

One of the insidious things about this disease is that you look ok, that no one knows how bad things are inside your body. How can life be so glorious, and the body so full of betrayal?

Even if you have the support and faith of those around you, there's a fear and despair that seems to accompany CFS and fibromyalgia that is not common in many other conditions.

You may feel as if the onset of your illness was a form of death, or at a minimum, a line that clearly divides your life into "before" and "after" CFS/fibromyalgia. Many people I talked to described these diseases as "monsters" they were battling. They described losing themselves and having pain and fatigue—both physical and emotional—that no one else except another sufferer seems to understand.

And as time goes on, it becomes clearer to you that many people simply won't understand. What do you say when someone asks you how you are?

Joyce explains the frustration:

It is a conundrum. I give mixed signals to others. Others who know me, whom I do not see frequently, but who know my condition ask me how I am. If I say good, fine with a cheerful voice they then make [the] assumption that I am better, and say "So you are better, you are over it?" Then I say no, that [it] is the same. And I wonder, do they think it odd or wrong for me to say fine? Can a quad in a wheelchair say she is fine? Of course, and no one expects her to get up from her wheelchair. When I say I am fine I have to explain more, and then the next question, "So they haven't figured out what it is yet?" As though if they had I would be better? Who ever gets better from chronic disabling conditions? People get worse or at best stabilize over time and it is considered just a tad indiscreet to ask someone with breast cancer, not cured, if they now have it in their bones. We don't do that. And yet with CFS there is this endless curiosity.

Bottom line?

I wrote this book to fast-forward you through the process that I've already gone through. If you had the energy and time, you could read the same fifty books and thousand research articles that I did, talk to dozens of experts, and correspond with thousands of fellow patients. But I guarantee you, if you did, you would come to the same conclusions that I did:

• You'll discover that there isn't a smoking gun—you won't find one particular trigger common to everyone who develops CFS or fibromyalgia. We're all different, and we develop CFS and/or fibromyalgia in different ways, for different reasons, as the result of different triggers.

• You'll see that there is no definitive list of guaranteed symptoms for either condition. There are some basic symptoms that are seen in many—but not all—patients, and many other symptoms that affect only some people. Your symptoms will likely be different from those of someone else with CFS or fibromyalgia. Everyone doesn't fit a mold, so your case of CFS or fibromyalgia may not resemble mine, and mine won't resemble the next person's.

• You'll find out that people get diagnosed in very different ways—and there's no single surefire way to get diagnosed. Your experience of getting diagnosed is likely to be quite different from mine. You may prefer to go the route of extensive testing. I may prefer to give my medical history, then move right into focusing on treatments, based on interpreting my history and symptoms.

• You'll find out that you can't find one particular type of doctor or specialty that is most likely to successfully diagnose or treat your CFS or fibromyalgia. The type of doctor who ultimately diagnoses you may not be able to diagnose me, and vice versa.

• And as for treatments, you'll learn that there isn't any over-the-counter supplement, prescription pill, surgery, or miracle cure-all that will easily and quickly restore you to good health. What actually works is an approach customized to each person's particular health situation.

It could sound bleak, but I assure you, it's truly not! Because you are reading this book.

And while there are no solutions that apply to everyone, there are effective solutions—but you have to find the unique combination that works for *you!*

I've put together the information you need to work out your own unique plan for living well. And I know the condition you are dealing with is quite real. And I know you're exhausted, and in pain, and I take it very seriously, because I've been there, too.

Creating your unique plan means you must be aware of and knowledgeable about your options, and fully prepared to participate in creating a plan for your own care and treatment. That is where *Living Well with Chronic Fatigue Syndrome and Fibromyalgia* will help.

While most books, organizations, and even physicians promote one particular theory and treatment approach, *Living Well with Chronic Fatigue Syndrome and Fibromyalgia* takes a look at the bigger picture, giving you the tools, resources, and information you need to create that personalized plan for living well with CFS or fibromyalgia. Tools and features include

- A detailed plan for getting diagnosed, including the tests you might ask for in some cases to aid in diagnosis
- Descriptions of risk factors and symptoms of CFS and fibromyalgia, and a comprehensive and detailed checklist you can use to aid in self-evaluation and diagnosis with your physician
- An overview of the various theories behind CFS and fibromyalgia—from infections, to hormone imbalances, to nervous system imbalances, to musculoskeletal problems, to sleep disorders, to nutritional deficiencies, and more. You can quickly become familiar with the many different schools of thought.
- Information to help you review and evaluate the many different options you can pursue in terms of treatment—from the most conventional therapies to the most alternative mind–body approaches
- A patient-oriented look at the popular protocols, including Dr. R. Paul St. Amand's "guai" protocol, Dr. Jacob Teitelbaum's interdisciplinary protocol, and more
- A look at the roles of hormonal treatments, antibiotic and antifungal treatments, dietary changes, detoxification, allergy treatment, stress reduction, attitude, lifestyle, mind, body, and spirit in treating fibromyalgia and CFS
- Detailed information on how to find and work with the right practitioners

- Guidelines on how to develop a comprehensive treatment plan
- A comprehensive Resources section with organizations, books, magazines, Web sites, and support groups that can help

It can be difficult, frightening, and frustrating to try to live well with CFS or fibromyalgia. But it can be done.

At the time when you need it most, this comprehensive guide will introduce you to these conditions, help you get diagnosed, and then provide you with the tools you need to carefully craft your own wellness plan and confidently carry it out with the aid of your practitioners.

■ My Own Story

Before I continue, I thought it might be useful to explain how I became so interested in CFS and fibromyalgia. To start, I'm not a doctor, and I'm not a health professional. I have an international business degree from Georgetown University, and a background in public relations and communications consulting. But along the way, my own frustrations with health care and efforts to live well were transformed into a career in patient advocacy and health writing.

My own health adventures actually began in December of 1978, when at seventeen years of age I had my first serious illness. I was in the midst of a busy, exciting few months of dating, working part-time, and attending the first half of my senior year of high school. Over the Christmas break, I came down with a terrible case of what seemed like bronchitis, but it quickly became clear that this was no ordinary bronchitis. I slept for ten-hour stretches, awaking only to take a sip of water, and then falling asleep again for hours.

After a trip to the doctor around the New Year, I was diagnosed with a particularly debilitating case of mononucleosis. My white count was so high that the doctor said it would be many months before I would recover and could return to school. He told my mother to plan for me to be in bed and out of school for the entire second half of the school year.

I was horrified. This was going to put quite a crimp in my plans for dating my steady boyfriend, going to our spring proms, graduating from high school, and getting ready to start college that fall. The doctor said there was absolutely nothing besides rest that could be done for my mono. The most exciting time of my life was turning into a total disaster.

My mother was determined to avoid disaster, however, and after consulting with a holistically minded friend, came home with a copy of Adele Davis's book *Let's Get Well*. The book included recommendations, including a host of vitamins and an antistress protein drink concoction to be taken multiple times a day, which it was claimed would help with mononucleosis. I took my vitamins and drink several times throughout each day and night, followed a high-protein diet, and rested. A week later, I felt my energy returning. Two weeks later, I felt almost normal. A trip to the doctor three weeks after diagnosis, along with a blood test, confirmed the good news. My skyrocketing white count had returned to normal. I was over my mononucleosis and could go back to school and resume my life!

My mother tried to tell my amazed doctor about our megavitamin approach. The doctor, a kindly but skeptical—and decidedly nonholistic—family doctor from the old school, wouldn't hear of it.

"I really don't want to know what you did, but whatever it is you think you did, it worked!" said the doctor.

I luckily enjoyed good health throughout my twenties, no thanks to me. I was slender, a coffee and cigarette addict who made do on five to six hours of sleep a night. I didn't exercise; I worked like a crazy person, and ate terribly, subsisting on red meat, potatoes, and junk food. I could go a week without encountering a vegetable.

I didn't give much thought to my health again until early 1993, when at the age of thirty-two, my body and I had a chance to get intimately reacquainted. At the time, I was working a very stressful full-time job where full-time was more like sixty hours a week. A few months earlier, my car had been rear-ended, and I was still experiencing neck and back pain. I was promoting my first book and would come home and then work into the wee hours of the morning. After a few hours of sleep, I'd wake up, and a few cups of coffee and cigarettes later, I was headed back to the office. I was starting an intense relationship with a new boyfriend. It was a period of about five months of working horrendously long hours, running on little sleep, and eating takeout and junk food, supplemented by plenty of cigarettes and caffeine.

I woke up one day with the worst bronchial infection I'd ever had. I felt as if I were going to die. In fact, secretly, I was certain I had some sort of horrendous disease no one had figured out yet, because I could barely lift an arm off the bed, much less get up and make my way to the bathroom.

All of a sudden, my life came to a grinding halt. No work, no book promotion, no dates—nothing. I was practically comatose on the sofa, unable to read, barely able to understand mindless television programs, and certain that I didn't even have the mental capacity to write a memo. I couldn't focus, could barely move, and on top of that, a numbing depression overtook me.

It took me weeks to even get the energy to go see the doctor, who ran a blood test and said that I had off-the-chart elevations of Epstein-Barr antibodies that indicated an active infection. And in the absence of anything else of note in my bloodwork, my doctor suggested that what was plaguing me looked like chronic fatigue syndrome.

Weeks dragged into months. Mail and laundry piled up. I had little appetite, but when I did manage to fix something, dirty dishes would sit for weeks in the sink.

And it was déjà vu. There I was again, at a time when things should have been going so well—new book, new boyfriend, exciting job—and I was practically flat on my back most of the time, exhausted, incapacitated, and depressed!

It was during this time that I realized my boyfriend would end up being my husband, because he stuck it out with me despite the fact that the new me was a disheveled, foggy, and depressed woman who had taken the place of the attractive, energetic, and sharp person I once was.

The lack of physical energy was hard, so hard, but what was even worse to me was what is called "brain fog," the inability to think clearly, the difficulty of putting together even a simple sentence, the frustration in trying to organize my thoughts. I was a person who made my living by writing, reading, and strategizing. And there I was, unable to imagine a day when I would feel well enough to be able to write a simple paragraph, much less return to work.

My doctor decided to try an aggressive program of acupuncture. She also recommended that I return to a diet and supplement program similar to the one I followed back when I had mononucleosis. She also had me eliminate all alcohol and caffeine from my diet.

Slowly, very slowly, I could feel energy returning. If I had to quantify it now, I would say that every month I felt maybe 1 or 2 percent better than the previous month. After a while, I felt well enough to return to work part-time, although for at least a year I felt slow and inefficient compared to my previous performance. I would plod through the workday feeling as if I were reading, thinking, and writing at half-speed, then come home from work and go to bed for twelve hours, until getting up for work the next day. I slept late into the day Saturdays and Sundays just to recuperate.

Eventually, I was back at work full-time, but still exhausted and fuzzy-brained most of the time. The weight started piling on as well, despite no change to my diet.

Months after my early 1995 wedding to the man who had stood by me, I was dealt another health blow. I was diagnosed with hypothyroidism caused by Hashimoto's thyroiditis, an autoimmune disease that had caused my thyroid to become underactive.

Despite having apparently "recuperated" from my nearly year-long bout with CFS, and being treated for the hypothyroidism, I still continued to develop all kinds of symptoms that mystified my doctor and me. My eyes became dry and gritty. My periods were heavier and more frequent. My skin started flaking. I had headaches. I had heart palpitations. My breathing felt heavy. I had excruciating pain in my ribs. My sides felt swollen. My hips ached, and there were spots in my neck and shoulder area that felt like someone had stabbed them with ice picks. My doctor sent me for second opinions from an infectious disease specialist, an endocrinologist, a physical therapist, a pulmonary specialist, a cardiologist, an internist, an ophthalmologist, and so on. I had MRIs, CT scans, ultrasounds, blood tests. I was poked and prodded, and my symptoms continued. Then came lower back pain, alternating diarrhea and constipation, and episodes of low blood sugar. I woke up multiple times per night for no apparent reason. Off I went for fasting glucose tests, stool analysis, an MRI of my back, and a prescription for sleeping pills.

Along the way, I had become dedicated to learning more about my thyroid condition, and ended up launching several Web sites and a newsletter, and ultimately, I wrote my first health book, *Living Well with Hypothyroidism*. As part of my research, I became familiar with the work of Dr. John Lowe, a fibromyalgia researcher, who suggested that there is a definite connection between hypothyroidism and fibromyalgia.

I asked my doctor to check my fibromyalgia trigger points, and sure enough, I had pain levels that went through the roof at nearly every single spot she tested. I met the criteria for a diagnosis of fibromyalgia, but my doctor and physical therapist didn't really think the official diagnosis was all that critical. Whether I had fibromyalgia or not, my doctor's recommended treatment was a combination of acupuncture, myofascial release physical therapy, thyroid hormone replacement, sleeping pills, and other dietary and lifestyle changes that I already had in progress.

Since that time, based on all my information gathering, I've changed my thyroid treatment, revised my supplement program dramatically based on what I learned, and have slowly started to incorporate Pilates—an exercise program that emphasizes abdominal and back strengthening—into my routine. I've changed my sleep patterns, and made a variety of other changes, including stress reduction and mind–body efforts. And I can say that today, as I write this, I am no longer in daily pain. My fibromyalgia trigger points are far less tender, I have almost no rib and lower back pain, and I manage to keep up a somewhat busy schedule on eight to nine hours of sleep a night. I'm living well.

So right now it appears that I'm not battling an active case of CFS or fibromyalgia. I couldn't be writing this book if I were, because at those times I was actively symptomatic, I was so exhausted that I could nod off in seconds while looking at a computer screen. I couldn't concentrate enough to put together a coherent paragraph. I would read the same few pages of a book or article over and over for hours, unable to absorb the meaning.

While not actively symptomatic, I am constantly on the alert for evidence that I am overdoing it, for even the earliest signs that my health is going to collapse on me, as it has done before, and launch me into an episode of CFS or fibromyalgia. I am like a thermostat, constantly monitoring my sleep, energy levels, and diet, and making adjustments every day. Some days I need to get extra sleep, others I slow down my exercise routine, add special supplements, or adjust the protein levels in my diet. The objective: to ward off any decline that could move me into chronic fatigue and body pain, and ultimately, back into full-scale CFS or fibromyalgia.

■ Moving Forward

My hope is that you move forward after reading this book with an understanding that *you* are the key to living well with CFS or fibromyalgia. You will need to trust your own instincts, find the right practitioner to be your partner in wellness, and use your own judgment to choose from among your options in terms of treatment.

I also hope that you will come away from this book aware of the many options—from prescription drugs, to vitamins, to supplements, to bodywork, to nutrition, and more—that can help with CFS and fibromyalgia. And I hope that armed with that knowledge, you'll be able to put it together, with the aid of your practitioner, into a plan that will work for you.

You deserve to live well.

2

Understanding Chronic Fatigue Syndrome and Fibromyalgia

You can't teach an old dogma new tricks.
—DOROTHY PARKER

To start, it's important to review chronic fatigue syndrome and fibromyalgia, the symptoms, and what we know about who and where they strike.

■ What Is Chronic Fatigue Syndrome?

Chronic fatigue syndrome is not like normal fatigue or exhaustion. The feeling has been likened to the fatigue and fuzzy-brained sensation of having a hangover or being in the worst stage of the flu, except it doesn't stop. Frequently, the fatigue comes on quickly, often accompanied by a bad sore throat, upper respiratory infection, cold, bronchitis, hepatitis, intestinal bug, food poisoning, mononucleosis, or intense stress. In some people, however, it begins slowly, with no apparent precipitating factor.

Officially, chronic fatigue syndrome (CFS)—which is sometimes also referred to as chronic fatigue immune dysfunction syndrome (CFIDS)—was defined in 1994 as: fatigue that is medically unexplained, of new onset, that lasts at least six months, that is not the result of ongoing exertion, that is not substantially relieved by rest, and that causes a substantial reduction in activity levels.

In addition to this extreme fatigue, for a diagnosis of CFS there must also be four or more of the following symptoms:

- Substantially impaired memory/concentration
- Sore throat
- Tender neck or armpit lymph nodes
- Muscle pain
- Headaches of a new type, pattern, or severity
- Unrefreshing sleep
- Relapse of symptoms after exercise (also known as postexertional malaise) that lasts more than twenty-four hours
- Pain in multiple joints without joint swelling or redness

In addition to the official defining symptoms of CFS, many other symptoms are reported, including abdominal pain, intolerance for alcohol and medications, bloating, chest pain, chronic cough, diarrhea, dizziness, dry eyes or mouth, earaches, irregular heartbeat and palpitations, nausea, night sweats, vertigo, panic attacks, shortness of breath, skin sensations, numbness and tingling, and weight changes, among others. A more extensive list of symptoms also associated with CFS is discussed in chapters 3 and 4. The above symptoms, however, constitute the criteria for official, conventional diagnosis of CFS.

While there is disagreement about the typical profile of the CFS patient, it's generally agreed that women are more likely to get CFS than men, and that the condition affects a higher percentage of those with lower incomes and has higher prevalence among African-Americans and Hispanics. But CFS is seen in all age ranges, from children to seniors, in all races, genders, ethnic groups, and economic levels.

From a demographic standpoint, the CFIDS Association of America has compiled a number of statistics regarding the condition:

- It's estimated that more than 800,000 people have CFS, and that estimate could be substantially higher due to the difficulty of identifying and diagnosing those CFS patients who are too sick to be evaluated.

- Less than 10 percent of CFS patients have been diagnosed and are receiving proper care for their disease.

- CFS is three times more common in women than men. The Centers for Disease Control (CDC) estimates that 522 women and 291 men are afflicted with CFS per 100,000 people.

- Among women, CFS is more common than multiple sclerosis, lupus, HIV infection, and lung cancer. CFS is a serious health concern when you consider that 522 women per 100,000 have the condition, compared to 12 per 100,000 with AIDS, 26 per 100,000 with breast cancer, 33 per 100,000 with lung cancer, 900 per 100,000 with diabetes, among other conditions.

- One research study found that CFS occurs in about 0.42 percent of the population, which is almost double the estimates made by the Centers for Disease Control.

- The highest risk agewise is among those forty to forty-nine.

There appears to be a genetic connection in CFS. One study showed that in identical twins where one has CFS, the other twin will also have it in 55 percent of cases. In fraternal twins where one has CFS, the other twin will have CFS 19 percent of the time. One study found that all offspring of twin pairs where only one twin has CFS were at increased risk of developing CFS. These family connections suggest some sort of a genetic role in the development of CFS.

A Condition by Any Other Name

Illnesses that resemble CFS have been reported as early as the 1800s, under different names. As early as 1860, CFS was referred to as neurasthenia by Dr. George Beard, who thought the condition was some form of nervous disorder, accompanied by weakness and fatigue.

In the early 1980s, CFS was referred to as the "yuppie flu," mainly because attention was focused on the affluent professional women in their thirties and forties who complained of the illness. It was thought that the disease was a form of burnout that affected overachievers with type A personalities. Interestingly, while it's been shown that the disease actually affects people from a range of age, race, economic level, and gender groups, this stereotype persists twenty years later.

After the "yuppie flu" period, the condition was frequently called "chronic Epstein-Barr virus" (CEBV), or "chronic mononucleosis," because doctors suspected some sort of connection between EBV—the virus that causes mononucleosis—and the onset of CFS. But when some CFS sufferers were found who did not have EBV antibodies, and it was shown that a high percentage of the population had EBV antibodies but did not develop CFS, this name also fell out of favor.

In the late 1980s, medical researchers interested in the syndrome worked with the CDC to first identify the symptom and physical criteria for diagnosis. At the time, they called the illness "chronic fatigue syndrome," given that the primary symptom was fatigue. In the United Kingdom and some other areas of the world, CFS is referred to as myalgic encephalomyelitis, or ME. Other common names for the condition include chronic fatigue and immune dysfunction syndrome (CFIDS), postinfectious neuromyasthenia and postviral fatigue syndrome.

A choice for an official name has been a major issue among advocates. There is a vocal contingent within the community of

CFS patients and practitioners who feel that the name "chronic fatigue syndrome" minimizes the attention to and seriousness of the condition. There is concern that despite being a prominent symptom, fatigue is not the main problem. Britain's CFS/ME working group report talked to patients, one of whom underscored that point, saying: "Alzheimer's disease is not known as 'Chronic Forgetfulness Syndrome.'"

Author and CFS patient Laura Hillenbrand, whose bestseller *Seabiscuit* topped the charts for months and was made into a documentary and a feature film, is another fan of a name change. She likes to quote another CFS patient, who told her: "Fatigue is to this illness as a match is to a nuclear bomb!"

In the U.S., in addition to CFS, chronic fatigue and immune dysfunction syndrome and chronic fatigue and immune dysregulation syndrome, both abbreviated as CFIDS, have been in use. But a survey of members of the CFIDS Association found that the majority still do not like the current name, and want the name changed as soon as possible.

In the United Kingdom, ME is favored as the choice for a new name for the condition throughout the medical community.

Overall, there is a strong sense that the name "chronic fatigue syndrome," by focusing on one symptom, encourages misunderstanding of the illness and contributes to the negative way in which patients and the disease are viewed. It's also clear that the name of the condition has contributed to less than optimal care in some environments. One interesting study found that greater time would be spent with a patient by physicians who were told the patient had myalgic encephalomyelitis versus chronic fatigue syndrome.

One patient, Roseanne, summed up the conflicting feelings very well:

"Chronic Fatigue Syndrome" is misleading. Not only is fatigue not the primary symptom for me now, it never has

been. For me, the illness I have is much more like AIDS, because of the dysfunctional immune system. It is hard for me to get rid of infectious illness. I have become increasingly sensitive to chemicals such as perfume, smoke, paint, and other household chemicals. Sometimes I board the bus, smell perfume, and have to get off at the next stop, and wait for the next one. This is NOT described by the words "Chronic Fatigue Syndrome," is it?

Another CFS patient, Cathy, agrees there should be a name change:

Can the name of your illness make you worse? "Chronic Fatigue Syndrome" is a terrible name for a disease. It suggests that [it] is only fatigue and that it is all in [the] mind. This is wrong on all counts. But the name itself encourages other people and authorities not to take this severely debilitating condition seriously, increasing the destructive isolation of sufferers.

The choice of a new name has been a difficult process, however. Names of some conditions focus on the cause of the condition, but since the cause is not clearly understood or known in CFS, that type of name is not an option. Other names often focus on symptoms, but since there are several key symptoms, this option can be difficult and unwieldy. There is general acceptance, however, that most symptoms are evidence of dysfunctions in the neurologic, neuroendocrine, and/or immunologic systems.

The U.S. Department of Health and Human Services CFS Coordinating Committee established the Name Change Workgroup (NCW) to propose a new name for CFS. After study and deliberation, the group is recommending that the name be changed to "neuroendocrineimmune dysfunction syndrome," or NDS. The group is recommending NDS as an umbrella term, to represent the broad range of CFS. The group also suggests that there be specific subgroups under the NDS umbrella, to enable more relevant research studies. The subgroups being recommended include

- NDS-Myalgic Encephalomyelitis
- NDS-Fukuda Criteria
- NDS-Canadian Clinical Criteria
- NDS-Gulf War syndrome/Gulf War Illness

NDS-Myalgic Encephalomyelitis (ME) refers to a condition that features extensive postexertional fatigue, central nervous system involvement such as sleep disorders, autonomic disturbances, cognitive problems, and a chronic nature, with relapses.

NDS-Fukuda refers to strict adherence to the CDC's criteria, which were defined by Dr. Fukuda and colleagues in 1994. The Fukuda criteria are used extensively as the official criteria for defining CFS around the globe. Some experts view the Fukuda criteria as too narrow by virtue of the fact that they exclude people who likely have the condition, but are excluded from diagnosis due to a medical history of medical and psychiatric conditions.

NDS-Canadian Clinical Criteria: A Canadian group has a definition that differs from the Fukuda criteria. The Canadian Clinical definition includes

- Six months' duration
- Significant new onset of unexplained, persistent, or recurrent physical or mental fatigue that substantially reduces activity level
- Postexertional malaise with loss of physical or mental stamina, rapid tiredness in muscles or cognitive ability, usually requiring twenty-four hours for recovery
- Unrefreshing sleep or sleep disturbance

- Significant muscle and joint pain
- Infectious illness onset while the patient has no pain or sleep dysfunction
- Two or more neurocognitive symptoms (such as confusion, difficulty concentrating, short-term memory problems)
- At least one symptom from two of the following categories: autonomic symptoms (neurally mediated hypotension, light-headedness), neuroendocrine symptoms (e.g., feeling of fever-ishness, cold extremities), and immune symptoms (e.g., recurrent sore throats)

NDS-Gulf War Syndrome: Gulf War Syndrome (GWS) is charac-terized by emphasis on primarily neurological symptoms involving the central, peripheral, and autonomic nervous systems. Symptoms include memory, thinking, attention problems, as well as sleep dis-turbances, fatigue depression, muscle and joint pains, fatigue, dizzi-ness, difficulty lifting, and numbness in the extremities.

Possible Causes/Triggers of CFS

Since intensive study has not found one particular precipitating factor, it's likely that CFS results from one or more of a variety of precipitating causes. Some of the theories behind the development of CFS and fibromyalgia include

INFECTIONS

- Viral infections, with enteroviruses such as Coxsackie virus, herpes viruses such as Epstein-Barr virus, cytomegalovirus, human herpes virus types 6 and 7, and herpes simplex virus types 1 and 2, stealth viruses, retroviruses, and other viruses
- Bacterial infection with chlamydia, mycoplasma, brucella, tick-borne bacterial conditions such as rickettsia, Lyme dis-ease, or Q fever

- Food-borne bacterial infection, including *Campylobacter jejuni*, shigella, *E. coli*, salmonella, cholera, *Clostridium botulinum*, *Yersinia enterocolitica*, *Listeria monocytogenes*, toxoplasma, and ciguatera
- Parasitic infections, including giardiasis, *E. histolytica*, *Cryptosporidium parvum*, *Cyclospora cayetanensis*, *Trichinella spiralis*, tapeworms, and flatworms
- Fungal infections, inluding chronic yeast/*Candida albicans* overgrowth

IMMUNE SYSTEM DYSFUNCTIONS
- Allergies
- Leaky gut
- Autoimmunity
- Th1/Th2 imbalance

HORMONAL, ENDOCRINE, AND HYPOTHALAMIC PITUITARY-ADRENAL (HPA) CONDITIONS
- Hypoadrenalism/adrenal insufficiency
- Hypothyroidism
- Growth hormone deficiency

CENTRAL NERVOUS SYSTEM AND CARDIAC DYSFUNCTION
- Neurochemical imbalances, i.e., low or blocked serotonin and endorphins, excess substance P, excess of NMDA (N-methyl-D-aspartate), blocked GABA (gamma-aminobutyric acid)
- Autonomic nervous system dysfunctions/dysautonomias, including postural orthostatic tachycardia syndrome (POTS), and neurally mediated hypotension (NMH)
- Heart problems, including cardiac viral infection and abnormal heart pumping

SENSITIVITIES, ALLERGIES, AND TOXIC EXPOSURES
- Chemical exposure
- Mercury/metals overexposure or toxicity
- Food allergies and sensitivities
- Neurotoxin exposure, including excitotoxins and ciguatoxin

NUTRITIONAL IMBALANCES OR DEFICIENCIES
- Deficiencies or imbalances in magnesium, l-carnitine, choline, B_{12}
- Phosphate excess, as postulated by R. Paul St. Amand, M.D., founder of the guaifenesin protocol

MUSCULOSKELETAL IMBALANCE/TRAUMA
- Whiplash and neck injury
- Brain stem area problems, including Chiari malformation

SLEEP DISORDERS & STRESS
- Sleep dysfunction, including stage 4/delta sleep dysfunction, insomnia, unrefreshing sleep, apnea, and myoclonus
- Stress response

The theory of infection opens up the possibility that the condition could be contagious. There were some cases of clusters of CFS outbreaks—for example, the famous early outbreak in Incline Village, Nevada, that suggested a possible infectious transmission mechanism. Conventional evaluation by the Centers for Disease Control, however, indicated that these outbreaks were not characterized as infectious. Some experts have suspected, however, that there could be an undetected or difficult-to-identify infectious agent, such as mycoplasma, or a stealth pathogen that is triggering CFS or involved in the outbreaks of CFS.

Diagnosis

There is no official test to diagnose CFS; rather it's a "diagnosis of exclusion," as other conditions that could account for the symptoms are ruled out.

Doctors typically perform a comprehensive medical history and physical exam. Blood and urine tests are performed to help rule out any other possible causes of the illness, including lupus, multiple sclerosis, Lyme disease, adrenal disorders, HIV or AIDS, thyroid disease, rheumatoid arthritis, depression, cancer, and other conditions.

If the doctor can identify no cause for the symptoms, then a diagnosis of CFS may be made.

Typical Course and Prognosis

It appears that the onset begins with some sort of triggering factor—either a physical or mental stressor, or some sort of infection. CFS can begin gradually or can come on very suddenly in an acute episode that most typically follows an acute infection, frequently viral.

The triggering factor then appears to cause a dysfunction in the immune system, and can reactivate latent viruses in some people. This leads to further immune dysfunction and resulting changes in the neuroendocrinological system. There is then an interaction between infection, immune dysfunction, and the neurohormonal and neuroendocrine abnormalities that appear to reinforce each other and manifest in varying symptoms.

Six weeks after the onset of the symptoms, a differential diagnosis of "acute fatigue syndrome" can be made. After three months, continuing symptoms can result in a provisional diagnosis of CFS, which can be confirmed at the six-month point.

The actual percentage of people who are considered "recovered" from CFS is not known.

Some patients will have partial recovery, with sufficient energy to return to some level of activity, but periodically experience episodes of CFS or CFS symptoms. Others have progressively worsening fatigue. And some patients will return to decent health and be free of CFS symptoms. According to the CDC, 50 percent of patients reported "recovery" (but again, keeping in mind that the definition of *recovery* may not have been complete freedom from symptoms), most often in the five years after onset of CFS.

Some studies on the prognosis of CFS have been among those who had the most severe and long-standing cases of CFS, which means that results tend to be skewed toward a poorer prognosis. One study has shown that children have the best outcomes, with 54 to 94 percent showing definite improvement in the six years after onset. From 20 to 50 percent of adults show some improvement, and 6 percent of adults return to the same level of functioning they had prior to onset.

Some studies are less optimistic, saying that no more than 5 to 10 percent of patients experience recovery. Others, however, offer a more optimistic interpretation. In one study of 155 CFS patients surveyed over a four- to eight-year period, 31 percent of patients described themselves as experiencing recovery during the first five years of illness, and 48 percent during the first ten years.

According to the CFIDS Association of America, physicians believe CFS is as disabling, or even more debilitating, than lupus, rheumatoid arthritis, and similar chronic conditions. Specifically, CFS can be categorized as mild, moderate, severe, or very severe:

• Mild CFS: Typically, if you have mild CFS, you're mobile, you can take care of yourself, you can perform some light physical tasks, you can usually still work, but you may need extra rest in order to be able to continue working.

• Moderate CFS: You're likely to have reduced mobility, you may not be able to perform your daily activities regularly, depending on your symptoms, you probably are not able to work, require extended rest periods, and may not be sleeping at night.

• Severe CFS: when CFS becomes severe, you may be able to perform only minimal daily tasks such as washing your face or brushing your teeth, you may have extreme difficulty with thinking and memory, and you may require a wheelchair.

• Very severe CFS: At this stage, a person is in bed most of the time and can't carry out daily tasks. It's estimated that as many as 25 percent of CFS patients may be so seriously affected that they can't perform basic tasks and may be almost entirely bedridden.

Treatments

Treatments for CFS range from a combination of antidepressants, sleep, and pain medications, to cognitive therapy, to a full range of alternative therapies, as outlined in this book. Conventionally, some physicians would say that there is no actual "treatment" for CFS. Since they don't really know what causes it, or what metabolic, immune, or infectious mechanism is at work to cause it, there's no specific treatment pinpointed, leaving conventional medicine somewhat at a loss for options and treatment more on a symptom-by-symptom basis.

■ What Is Fibromyalgia?

Fibromyalgia (pronounced fy-bro-my-AL-ja) is a chronic condition characterized by widespread musculoskeletal pain, fatigue, and multiple tender points.

The word *fibromyalgia* is derived from the Latin: "fibro" (supportive, fibrous tissue such as ligaments, tendons, or fascia), "myo" (muscle), and "algia" (pain). Fibromyalgia is also sometimes referred to as fibrositis or fibromyositis.

Fibromyalgia (also called FMS, for fibromyalgia syndrome) can be quite difficult to diagnose because it shares symptoms with many other disorders.

According to the American College of Rheumatology (ACR)'s 1990 criteria for classifying fibromyalgia, a person is considered to have fibromyalgia if he or she has widespread pain for at least three months in combination with tenderness in at least eleven of eighteen specific tender point sites.

Pain is considered widespread when it occurs in both the left side of the body and the right side, and both above and below the waist. Cervical spine, anterior chest, thoracic spine, or low back pain must also be present.

The "tender points" are precise areas of the body which, when pressed, generate pain. The eighteen tender point sites:

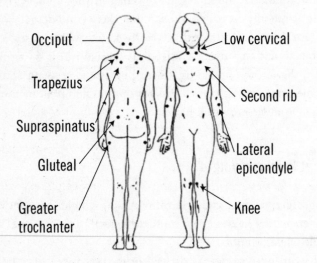

1. The area where the neck muscles attach to the base of the skull, left and right sides (occiput)

2. Midway between neck and shoulder, left and right sides (trapezius)
3. Muscles over left and right upper inner shoulder blade, left and right sides (supraspinatus)
4. Two centimeters below side bone at elbow of left and right arms (lateral epicondyle)
5. Left and right upper outer buttocks (gluteal)
6. Left and right hip bones (greater trochanter)
7. Just above left and right knees on inside
8. Lower neck in front, left and right sides (low cervical)
9. Edge of upper breastbone, left and right sides (second rib)

To be considered painful, pressure on the tender point must generate actual pain, not just tenderness.

Though not part of the official diagnosis, people with this syndrome may also experience sleep disturbances, morning stiffness, irritable bowel syndrome, anxiety, and other symptoms.

According to the American College of Rheumatology, fibromyalgia affects three to six million Americans. Fibromyalgia primarily occurs in women of childbearing age, but children, the elderly, and men can also be affected. FMS in children may be more common than assumed, however. One study found that among healthy schoolchildren, as many as 6 percent met fibromyalgia criteria.

About 90 percent of all people with fibromyalgia are women, 10 percent men. In general, fibromyalgia strikes women seven times more often than men, according to a 1998 National Institutes of Health report.

Fibromyalgia is more than twice as common as rheumatoid arthritis.

Possible Causes/Triggers of Fibromyalgia

The cause of fibromyalgia is not known, but researchers have a number of theories about what causes or triggers the condition. In addition to sharing many of the same trigger theories as CFS, some of the theories regarding fibromyalgia include

- Injury or trauma that affects the musculoskeletal system
- Injury or trauma that affects the nervous system
- Changes in muscle metabolism that cause fatigue and decreased strength
- Profound sleep dysfunction
- Response to an infectious agent, such as a virus or bacteria
- Hypometabolism, an underactive thyroid, or thyroid hormone resistance
- Post-traumatic stress

Diagnosis

Unfortunately, no medical test or X-ray can provide a definitive diagnosis of fibromyalgia.

Doctors typically use the American College of Rheumatology criteria described earlier for physical evaluation and diagnosis.

There are some blood work findings that may help in a diagnosis, including low serotonin levels, elevated levels of substance P, low levels of adenosine triphosphate (ATP), low free cortisol levels in twenty-four-hour urine testing, hypoglycemia, and low levels of growth hormone. But frequently the tests are not conducted, and a diagnosis is made based on physical examination.

Typical Course and Prognosis

In fibromyalgia it appears that there is a similar model to CFS as far as the typical course, with some variations.

Something appears to trigger FMS, and perhaps while infection may not be as prevalent a trigger as in CFS, physical or emotional traumas appear to be factors as well. In particular, trauma to the neck—whiplash, for example—appears to be connected to the onset of fibromyalgia in some patients.

The triggering factor then appears to cause a dysfunction in the immune system and/or the neurological system and pain receptors. This leads to further immune dysfunction and resulting changes in the neuroendocrinological system. There is again an interaction between infection, immune dysfunction, and the neurohormonal and neuroendocrine abnormalities that appear to reinforce each other and manifest in varying symptoms.

An official diagnosis of fibromyalgia can be made after three months of widespread pain, and for many practitioners, fulfillment of the ACR criteria.

The prognosis for fibromyalgia patients seems to depend on the research study you read.

Some studies have shown that most fibromyalgia patients experience little improvement in symptoms, but that over time, ability to cope with symptoms and pain becomes better, resulting in somewhat improved quality of life.

Other studies show that there can be remissions in as many as 24 percent of patients, and symptom improvement in almost half of all patients.

Treatment

Much as with CFS, there is no agreed-upon standard, proven "treatment" for fibromyalgia. Rather there is a collection of various approaches that address different symptoms, each approach having varying levels of success with each fibromyalgia patient. These approaches typically focus on pain relief, sleep improvement, and some form of stretching or exercise, and are discussed at length in subsequent chapters here in the book.

■ Viewing Chronic Fatigue Syndrome and Fibromyalgia Together

Some will strongly disagree that CFS and fibromyalgia can or should be viewed through the same lens, the approach I have taken in this book. They argue that "lumping" the two conditions together and broadening the definitions encourage researchers to do the same, making it difficult or impossible to conduct substantive, detailed research on the specific conditions. There is also a position that viewing CFS and fibromyalgia as similar conditions or in the same category of illness results in research that provides conflicting—and therefore practically useless—results.

Others suggest that the similarities between the conditions cannot be denied. Some research has found that as many as 70 percent of those with CFS meet the criteria for fibromyalgia, and up to 70 percent of patients with fibromyalgia meet the criteria for CFS. This suggests that the conditions may share similar causes, paths, and results for many patients, and that these similarities suggest that a more integrative treatment approach be taken.

Still others, such as Dr. John Lowe of the Fibromyalgia Research Foundation, believe that CFS and fibromyalgia are in fact the same condition with the same basic cause, with the main difference being the dominant symptom, fatigue versus pain.

According to Craig Maupin, a CFS patient advocate and author of *The CFIDS Report,* some of the confusion may be due to the fact that we could view CFS as really two different conditions:

- The classic CDC-criteria type of CFS that is characterized by flulike symptoms, infectious onset, extreme fatigue, activity intolerance, major debilitation, and poor prognosis

and

- CFS that is similar to fibromyalgia, does not feature exercise intolerance as a key feature, and can be improved by graded exercise

According to Maupin, researchers have found an immune defect in those patients in the first group that is not seen in fibromyalgia patients or health control subjects. This finding may argue for a separation in the view and treatment of CFS and fibromyalgia.

Differences

There are some very definite differences between CFS and fibromyalgia. Just a few of note include the following:

- CFS is diagnosed by excluding and ruling out all other conditions; fibromyalgia is diagnosed using the American College Rheumatology criteria and trigger point tests.
- Fibromyalgia is far more prevalent than CFS.
- The primary symptom in CFS is considered the extreme fatigue that is so debilitating that even a minimal exertion can leave someone bedridden. Fibromyalgia's main symptom is considered to be severe body pain.
- CFS patients have a strong intolerance for exercise, while fibromyalgia patients may find exercise therapeutic and helpful in many cases.
- Two symptoms unique to CFS and not frequently seen in fibromyalgia are mild fever or chills and sore throat.
- Unique to fibromyalgia and not frequently seen in CFS is pain, especially lower back pain, that is improved by heat or massage and worsened by standing or sitting.
- CFS patients more often have abnormal changes in the blood flow to the brain, as seen in SPECT (single photon emission computerized tomography) and PET (positron emission tomography)

analysis, BEAM (brain electrical activity mapping), and MRI (magnetic resonance imaging). These changes are not seen as frequently in fibromyalgia.

Similarities

Both CFS and fibromyalgia are most prevalent in women in the twenty-to-fifty-year-old-age range. A number of symptoms appear to be common to most people with CFS or fibromyalgia:

- Muscle pain, aching, weakness
- Sleep disturbances and unrefreshing sleep
- "Brain fog"—memory problems, confusion, poor concentration
- Abdominal pain
- Hard, loose, or watery stools
- Fatigue, including postexertional fatigue in some cases
- Headaches
- Joint pain without redness or swelling

Fever, swollen glands, and cognitive dysfunction are seen in both conditions, but are far more common in chronic fatigue patients. And irritable bowel syndrome, premenstrual flares, and vulvodynia (pain in the vaginal area) are seen in both conditions, but are far more common in fibromyalgia patients.

■ Moving Forward

Because of the similarities and overlap, and the theoretical idea on the part of some practitioners that the conditions may be facets of the same as yet understood malfunction, I felt it would be appropriate to bring the two conditions together into one book and view them through the same general lens. I hope this combined approach can be of particular help to those many patients who have overlapping symptoms of both conditions, those who are struggling to get a diagnosis, or the many who actually are diagnosed with both conditions.

3

Risk Factors and Symptoms

Lord, grant me the serenity to accept the things I cannot change,
the courage to change the things I can,
and the wisdom to hide the bodies of
doctors I shot when they said,
"You're perfectly healthy, it's all in your head."
—ANONYMOUS

There are a variety of well-accepted factors that can potentially increase the risk of developing CFS and/or fibromyalgia. In addition, there are markers—including a past history of certain medical conditions—that also may put you at a higher risk of developing these conditions. And a variety of symptoms can point to a diagnosis of CFS, fibromyalgia, or both. While some of the information is research based, some is anecdotal information that has come from practitioners and patients. This chapter discusses the risk factors, markers, and symptoms of these conditions, and describes them in more detail, including the words of real patients who are struggling with the symptoms every day.

Chapter 4 features a detailed checklist of these risk factors, markers, and symptoms that you can copy and take to your doctor to provide specific details on your health, and to aid in diagnosis and treatment of symptoms.

■ Risk Factors/Markers

Gender
Being female means that your risk for CFS or fibromyalgia is higher, in all age groups.

Family History
A family history of CFS or fibromyalgia means that you are at some increased risk for the condition. The specific risk is not known, since there are environmental factors, in addition to genetics, that drive the development of these conditions.

Medical History
Having a family or personal history of certain other conditions puts you at increased risk for CFS and fibromyalgia. Such conditions include

- Irritable bowel syndrome (IBS)
- Endometriosis
- Thyroid disease—hypothyroidism, hyperthyroidism
- Mood disorder
- Chronic or persistent nasal symptoms/sinusitis/sinus infections
- Ear infections (particularly with CFS)
- Hysterectomy (particularly with CFS)
- Miscarriage
- Irregular menstrual cycle
- Ovarian cysts

- Mononucleosis/glandular fever
- Epstein-Barr virus

Recent Infection

Having had a recent infection is a risk factor for both conditions, particularly for CFS. Some researchers claim that at least 10 percent of cases of CFS start after infection. The most commonly cited infections include

- Mononucleosis/glandular fever
- Epstein-Barr virus
- Viral meningitis
- Viral hepatitis
- Herpes
- Enteroviruses
- Hepatitis
- Salmonella
- Toxoplasmosis
- Influenza

Clara feels that her case of CFS (she is from the United Kingdom and calls it myalgic encephalomyelitis or ME) developed after an infection.

I was at University myself when I was first struck down with ME. In a sentence: I caught the flu and my life was never to be the same again. Of course, I didn't know that at the time. It was easily the worst flu I ever had in my life, but I presumed that was all it was, until it didn't go away. I would feel slightly better for a few days and then 'wham'! It was like being hit by a juggernaut all over again. My GP ran blood tests and identified a virus called Coxsackie. I was told to be careful, take rest as I needed it, and apparently the virus would burn itself out. I tried to carry on as normal but after just a few weeks I returned to my parents' house at the point of collapse. Rapidly I developed new symptoms. Symptoms I had never even heard of, or thought possible. I was bed bound and when I tried to sit up I felt as if my brain was slopping around in a solution inside my skull. Light stung my eyes and I developed visual disturbances: fluorescent green afterimages and strobe like flickering in my peripheral vision. By now I was too weak to stand up in the shower or wash my own hair. I was referred to a specialist for infectious diseases . . . after checking me over he made a diagnosis of ME.

Nancy also felt that her condition began with some sort of infection.

I woke that morning feeling fragile, perhaps coming down with flu. The walk from the bus stop to my office building was an exercise in tenacity, one foot in front of the other, don't stop, keep breathing. Collapsed in my chair, staring at my computer screen, all I could think of was the coming long weekend—three days in which to recoup my strength. The rest of that day passed in a haze. At noon I rested my head on my desk and fell into a coma-like sleep that left me disoriented and woozy. Finally 4:00 pm rolled around. It was a slight uphill walk to the bus stop but it might as well have been Mt. Everest. By the time I reached the corner, I was gasping for air and trembling as if I had just completed a marathon. I'm still not sure how I managed to endure the 50-minute bus ride home. My husband took one look at me and headed to the local emergency ward. I spent five hours there, enduring a multitude of tests, leaving with a vague diagnosis and a sinking feeling that this was not going to be over quickly.

Autoimmune Disease History

Some experts believe that having a family or personal history of autoimmune disease puts you at increased risk of CFS or fibromyalgia because they classify these conditions as autoimmune. Some of the more common autoimmune diseases include Hashimoto's thyroiditis, Graves' disease, rheumatoid arthritis, type 1 diabetes, multiple sclerosis, vitiligo, scleroderma, psoriasis, lupus, and Sjögren's syndrome.

Physical Injuries/Trauma

Physical injuries and physical trauma are risk factors for both conditions, but are more likely to trigger fibromyalgia. In particular, whiplash is one trauma associated with increased risk of fibromyalgia.

Fiona's health issues began when she had a serious car accident in May of 2000.

The other driver hit my car in the left rear side causing the car to spin completely around, hit a light pole, cause the pole to fall on the back of the car. I was wearing my seat belt and my Honda has a headrest; I feel both those factors minimized the damage to my neck. My body was bruised from the left shoulder to the right hip, or where I had pressed against the seat belt. I was taken by ambulance to the ER where I was monitored for damage to the heart and lungs due to the impact of the crash on my chest. I was given pain medication and sent home to rest. I took the pain medication and slept constantly for a few days. My eyes were hurting so I was driven to see the ophthalmologist, he noted that the lining of the eyes was detached, fortunately there was no retinal tear, but the doctor is still monitoring me closely. I soon realized I was paralyzed with the fear of getting into another car even as a passenger, since the other driver had hit my car as I was driving through an intersection with the green light. I felt I had no control of the other cars on the road and could fall victim again. I was also concerned with my loss of vision and income. In short order I became very depressed and while being treated, the depression lingered throughout the summer. As did the pain in my hips, knees, hands, shoulders and neck, unfortunately the pain grew in intensity in all those areas, prompting my rheumatologist to check all 18 fibromyalgia points. He found tenderness in every point and said I had fibromyalgia.

Hypermobile Joints

One potential risk factor or marker for CFS, according to experts from the Johns Hopkins Children's Center, is hypermobility of joints. Among those children and teenagers who had been treated for CFS, Johns Hopkins's experts found that 60 percent had hypermobility in at least four joints. Hypermobility is unusual flexibility in a joint— such as being able to bend your pinkie 90 degrees backward, touch your thumb to your forearm, or touch palms flat on the floor without bending your knees, and is seen in only 20 percent of the general population. The experts suspect that these hypermobile joints may put added stress on the nervous system, contributing to the risk.

Toxic Exposures

Sometimes referred to as "toxicant-induced loss of tolerance" ("TILT"), or defined as multiple chemical sensitivity, chronic exposure, overexposure, or in some cases even a one-time exposure to various toxins can in some cases trigger CFS or fibromyalgia. Some of the toxins implicated include herbicides, pesticides, insecticides, solvents, traffic exhaust, fragrances, gasoline, floor polish, copy machines, carpet cleaner, new carpets, adhesives, paints and spray paints, flame retardants, and many other common products. Metals are also implicated, including mercury, lead, cadmium, arsenic, aluminum, nickel, silver, beryllium, and tin.

Severe Life Stress

A history of severe life stress is more common in patients with both CFS and fibromyalgia.

Type A Personality

While it's controversial, some experts and patients believe that having a Type A personality or being a particularly driven high achiever may put you at more risk for CFS or fibromyalgia.

Marla describes how she was prior to her illness.

"Before," as we say, I was very much a Type A personality. I was successful in my work in upper management, an enthusiastic contributor to my community, a person who could and liked to do ten things (very well, I must say) at once.

Recent Immunizations/Vaccinations

Recent immunization or vaccination is a risk factor for both conditions, in particular CFS.

Medications/Drugs

Use of a variety of prescription medications has been associated with the onset of CFS. A partial list of the drugs include

Accutane	Ergamisol
Buspar	Lariam
Cordarone	Lopressor
Depo-Provera	Neupogen
Desyrel	NORVASC
Epogen	Parlodel

Prinivil

Procardia

Procrit

Prozac

Reglan

Tenormin

Toprol

Wellbutrin

Xanax

Zestril

Zoloft

■ Symptoms

CFS Symptoms—Official Criteria

To review, the official criteria for CFS include the following symptoms:

Fatigue that is medically unexplained, of new onset, that lasts at least six months, that is not the result of ongoing exertion, that is not substantially relieved by rest, and that causes a substantial reduction in activity levels.

Plus four or more of the following symptoms:

- Substantially impaired memory/concentration
- Sore throat
- Tender neck or armpit lymph nodes
- Muscle pain
- Headaches of a new type, pattern, or severity
- Unrefreshing sleep
- Relapse of symptoms after exercise (also known as postexertional malaise) that lasts more than twenty-four hours
- Pain in multiple joints without joint swelling or redness

Fibromyalgia Symptoms—Official Criteria

The official American College of Rheumatology criteria for fibromyalgia include

• Widespread pain for at least three months. Pain should be on both the left side of the body and the right side, and both above and below the waist. Cervical spine, anterior chest, thoracic spine, or low back pain must also be present.

• Pain in at least eleven of eighteen specific tender point sites, which were discussed in the previous chapter.

Pain, Aches, Stiffness

The pain of CFS, and fibromyalgia in particular, is a debilitating symptom for many people. Pain can strike almost any part of the body, from the head to the feet, in muscles (where it is known as myalgia) and joints (where it is known as arthralgia). The pain can be stationary, or it can move, but the most characteristic aspect of the pain is the intensity. Most people who experience the pain of fibromyalgia or CFS describe it as being unlike any other pain. The pain can be so intense that even a light touch is excruciating, or the weight of a handbag on a shoulder is unbearable. Pain can range from stiffness to aching, to soreness, to burning, to full shooting, stabbing pains.

Caroline, a woman with fibromyalgia, describes the pain she experienced.

I kept getting pain in my neck and it was always so stiff. Then I would get headaches, and pain in the back of my shoulder blades—pain that I cannot even describe. I never knew what pain was until the fibromyalgia. My fingers get stiff, I feel needles on the bottom of my feet, my neck stiffens up where I cannot move it, my hips hurt, I get swollen up, never a day or minute without pain. I have a lot of limitations. My mind says yes my body says no.

Julia describes her experience with fibromyalgia pain:

Four years ago I had been in a very minor car accident. The next day we drove to Florida. The car ride down there was uneventful, but during our one-week vacation, at times I was not able to hold my purse because the pressure on my neck and shoulders was too much. I treated pain with Aleve, which helped sometimes. The ride home a week later was painful to the point of extreme emotional and physical pain in my neck, shoulders and arms. When I got home I went to the chiropractor in the town where I work to see if he could help me. His first session did give me relief, but it was down hill after that. By my third visit he could not touch me anywhere, even a light massage, without excruciating pain. I had never heard of fibromyalgia, but he suggested that I have an evaluation by my internist because I had tenderness in 16 of the 19 pressure points.

Krista's fibromyalgia pain is worst at night.

I HATE nighttime as I hurt the most when my body is mobile . . . I hate the silence of the night . . . I can almost hear the pain as well as feel it in my body. Fibromyalgia seems to move from muscle to muscle . . . depending on what you have done, where you have done it and how you have done it. Some months my legs are bad . . . some months my arms are bad . . . some months my back is bad . . .

Pat feels that people don't understand the nature of the pain.

Most people do not understand about fibromyalgia and how debilitating the pain is. It's constant pain that never goes away. It just wears a person down.

Muscles

Muscles are frequently involved in CFS and fibromyalgia. Some people experience near-paralyzing muscle weakness (known as paresis) that is so severe that it's difficult or impossible to get out of bed or walk. Muscles can also cramp, twitch, or spasm in areas around the body, from eye twitches to twitches in arms and legs.

Headaches

Headache pain is a symptom in both CFS and fibromyalgia. There are two types of headache that are most often seen in CFS and fibromyalgia:

• Recurrent tension headaches. These are tension headaches that usually involve contraction of the muscles in the head, neck, and shoulders, will feel like a tight band around the head, frequently affecting the jaw, forehead, temple, or back of the neck.

• Recurrent migraine headaches. Migraines are frequently one-sided and accompanied by sensitivity to light, a pounding sensation, nausea, vomiting, visual disturbances, and dizziness.

Clara describes the kind of headaches she experienced with CFS:

The pain in my head lasted the better part of 3 years without a moment's relief. No painkillers touched it and I only vomited the stronger ones back up. I remember banging my head against the wall above my bed to see if that would help. I felt as if my whole brain had been burnt by a blowtorch and I repeatedly imagined myself opening my skull and pouring iced water over those cauliflower grooves of gray matter.

Fatigue

Fatigue is one of the most debilitating symptoms for people with CFS and/or fibromyalgia. But when we say "fatigue," we are not talking about the normal type of fatigue that people feel after a workout session, a poor night's sleep, or long hours at the office for a few days. This fatigue is more of an extreme exhaustion, the kind of fatigue that disrupts your life even when getting plenty of sleep, and interferes with your normal level of activities. This is fatigue that doesn't improve, even after sleeping twelve hours. If you can imagine the worst fatigue you ever felt in the midst of the flu, and multiply by it by 100, this is the type of fatigue that some people feel every single day with CFS or fibromyalgia.

Lynn describes the fatigue that plagues her:

I sometimes wonder if maybe I am just plain lazy because I want to sleep so much, or because I don't feel like vacuuming, cooking, cleaning, talking, or engaging in any activity whatsoever. Then I remember when this first hit me. I started getting sore muscles that I initially attributed to exercise. I became so tired that I thought I had a flu that simply wouldn't leave. I used to run. I ran all through middle and high school and into my 30's. I cannot run now. I try to move quickly to be the way I used to be; clean my whole house in 2 hours and then cook, shop, etc., and have time to spend having fun with my kids. I cannot clean for more than 30 minutes without complete exhaustion. Nor can I cook or shop for hours either, like I always used to do. The short time it takes me to make a meal causes me to be so uncomfortable that I cannot even think about eating it. I feel like my body has betrayed me. I am not lazy; I just have this illness that many doctors don't even recognize as being real. I WANT to run, clean my house, cook, dance, stay out past 8:00 pm without feeling sick, and just enjoy my kids. It's not that I don't want to. I can't.

Colleen, a teenager with CFS, describes her fatigue:

Most teenagers spend their days laughing and having fun. On the weekends, they go to football games, or out to the movies. I couldn't even make it to school. Instead of dates with a new boyfriend, I had doctors' visits. Instead of the movies, I had to rest. Some teens run track in high school. I couldn't even make it up a flight of stairs without being exhausted.

Rena describes her fatigue as "a world void of energy." Says Rena:

A trip from the living room sofa to the bathroom down the hall feels like a 5-mile hike in the woods.

Cate says that it's hard to explain the fatigue and pain to others because

I look healthy. When I told one friend that I had been diagnosed with fibro, she said, "oh yeah, that's that made-up disease, isn't it?" I'm depressed because I'm always so tired and tired because I'm always depressed.

Exercise and Exertion Intolerance

A particular type of fatigue that is seen in CFS and fibromyalgia patients is postexertional fatigue or malaise, or what's also known as exercise intolerance. This typically involves muscle pain and exhaustion after exercise, often going on as long as twenty-four hours or more. Some people have a delayed-reaction postexertional fatigue, and the fatigue will come on two to three days after physical exertion. Others have a full relapse of their symptoms, not just fatigue, after exercise or exertion.

Jeanne describes her experience:

I had been a regular swimmer, swimming 32 laps every other day. I was suddenly unable to swim more than 8 laps and felt winded, unwell and ached all over for the next several days as well as feeling in general worse for several days. . . . It would be so easy to dream that I might just break free of it for an hour and run, and climb a mountain, or a hill—exert myself without caution and feel tired, have sore muscles—that good kind of tired, where one become[s] rejuvenated by some hot chocolate, and a warm bath. Instead, every action must be calculated. If I do this now, then I must have time to rest before I can do that. If I want to go out tonight I must organize my day just so to improve the odds that I will be up for it later. And then, if I suddenly crash, that too I need to respect and respond to by canceling my plans. It takes a kind of patience and persistence that has to be continually rejuvenated.

Jessica describes the experience as "constantly recovering from the day before." Says Jessica:

I awake exhausted, my body hurts and I stretch and hardly have the energy to go further into the day. I am so tired of being sick. I feel like I am losing my driving force and motivation in life. CFS can suck it out of you. When I think of myself as a phoenix rising, I find that the pile is still burning itself, the supposed ashes, and it still finds tinder. The phoenix keeps getting burned again and again, never rising fully. I wonder how much of myself I have to let go before I can begin again. I think that I've let it all go and then there's more. I am tired.

Sleep Disturbances

Sleep disturbances are one of the most common features of CFS and fibromyalgia. There are a variety of ways that sleep is disturbed. Some people experience morning fog (or what's known as dysania), which is a feeling of being between asleep and awake. This can require that you stay in bed for an hour or two after waking in order to feel clear and awake enough to get out of bed. Some people experience sleep myoclonus or restless leg syndrome, with nighttime jerking, jumping, and spasming of arms and legs, or a feeling of itchiness or crawly sensations on the legs at night. One of the most characteristic symptoms is "unrefreshing sleep"—waking up feeling as if you hadn't slept, sometimes more tired than when you went to bed. Others can't fall asleep in the first place, wake frequently when they do fall asleep, have trouble falling back asleep after waking or frequent nighttime urination, or they wake too early and can't fall back asleep. Night sweats are also a problem for some.

Rita describes her sleep problems:

I was involved in a car accident in June 1998. The accident triggered a depressive episode that was recognized by a therapist approximately one year after the accident. I then sought the services of a psychiatrist. As I was being treated for the depression, the depressive symptoms were silently and gradually being replaced by those of fibromyalgia. I first noticed that something was terribly wrong when I consistently awoke in the morning feeling just as tired as when I went to sleep the night before. The quality of my sleep had changed from the early awakening, characteristic of depression to an awakening that felt unrefreshed with body-wide aches and pains—as if I hadn't slept at all! This was not at all like the depressive symptoms I had experienced and was not at all "normal" for me, a type A individual who prided herself on being driven to get things done, with energy to spare.

Breathing/Respiratory/Nose/Throat

The respiratory system seems to be an area for symptoms in CFS and fibromyalgia. Symptoms can range from shallow breathing and shortness of breath to sinus problems, stuffy or congested nose, trouble swallowing, and, more commonly in CFS, a sore throat.

Cognitive/Thinking/Memory/Concentration

Cognitive disturbances—difficulty with thinking, memory, and concentration—are among the most troublesome symptoms of CFS and fibromyalgia. Sometimes referred to as "brain fog," or as "fibro-fog" by fibromyalgia patients, the cognitive problems can really span a variety of symptoms. Some people have difficulty concentrating, a poor attention span, difficulty learning, a bad memory, and are easily distracted.

In some cases, people have more severe short-term memory problems, such as an inability to remember what they went to the store to buy, or confusion such as difficulty remembering familiar faces, locations, or directions. Some people describe word confusion or word substitution, difficulty finding the right word, reversing word order, or reversing first letter and sounds (known as pseudodyslexia). Math seems to present particular problems to some, whether it's addition or remembering a phone number.

Brad describes the problems his ten-year-old daughter faced when she was diagnosed with CFS.

She had a sledding accident with facial injuries when she was 9 followed by a viral illness that lasted several weeks. She appeared to have recovered from both but the CFS hit several months later and did not go away. My daughter has been so ill that she has missed almost two years of school. In addition to the terrible exhaustion, there is significant and constant pain (in her case headache and neck and upper back pain).

She has also had dizziness and postural orthostatic intolerance, tender lymph nodes, sore throat, sensitivity to sound and light, and sleep disruption. However, one of the greatest hardships has been the devastating change in her ability to learn. She was one of the brightest students in her class but now, cannot calculate (add, subtract, divide, multiply) at all. She has tremendous difficulty writing and has much more trouble remembering and processing information. This is often described as cognitive disruption but in severe cases like hers, makes getting back to normal school and activities extremely challenging.

Jessie describes the frustrations she deals with regularly:

I feel like I am treading water, like I am stuck in one place and not going anywhere. I want to use my brain more, but I am not sure how. I can't read much or focus at all. I forget words and can't fathom complex paragraphs. I love my life, but I feel like my brain is missing. When faced with a whole day, I can't see what I can accomplish with the tiny amount of energy I have. Today I am feeling a real loss of self as worker, intellectual, social being. I feel like I am oblivious all the time during conversations, and pass through interactions without taking note.

Laura has a funny anecdote to share about her brain fog:

One day at work when I had been particularly stressed out and in pain, I called my husband Tom at home to let him know what I thought we should have for dinner that night (he had called earlier to ask my opinion). I managed to dial the correct phone number after only one try, and the answer-

ing machine picked up. So far so good, I thought, then confidently gave my little message about supper, beginning with the unforgettable introduction: Hello, Laura, this is Tom!

Annie brings up one of the key problems for people with CFS or fibromyalgia—the difficulty understanding a complicated condition when one of the symptoms itself is brain fog.

Some hospital workers have assumed that my inability to convince them of my claims with lots of proof while lying in a hospital bed is evidence that my illness isn't real. The sicker I am, the harder it is for me to organize my thoughts sufficiently to present a good argument.

Connie, who was an intensive care nurse before her fibromyalgia was diagnosed, describes her cognitive symptoms:

The damage is permanent; I have altered brain chemistry. It doesn't show except in those very subtle ways; a certain lack of balance, an inability to find the right word sometimes, a tendency to run into things, or to drop things, blurred vision that makes it difficult to recognize people on bad days, and impossible to read, a painful sensitivity to light and sound, or too much activity around me. . . . The symptoms come and go without warning . . . all of which make me seem 'strange' to people I would otherwise expect to be supportive.

Mood/Depression

Changes in mood, the blues, anxiety, and feelings of depression are quite common in both CFS and fibromyalgia. Some people also notice more intense seasonal blues, with increased depression, irritability, and sleep disturbances in fall and winter, with some improvement in the spring and summer, sometimes referred to as seasonal affective disorder (SAD).

Lorraine describes her experience with depression, and why it's a problem for many people with CFS or fibromyalgia:

> *Some people think depression causes fibromyalgia, when in actuality fibromyalgia is the cause of our depression. Being in constant pain, which varies in intensity on a daily basis, flaring up for many different reasons or for no apparent reason at all, has made this woman whom [sic] was once a strong and independent individual, depressed. So, yes, people with fibro are depressed but it's because of having this chronic illness.*

Carmela, who has both fibromyalgia and CFS, asks some telling questions about the depression:

> *What are these monsters that can cause so much pain, fatigue and depression? Makes you feel like you need to be in the hospital, hooked up to a morphine pump, and being taken care of! We complain for a few years, but, no one listens, we look fine. So we hide our pain, anger, fatigue, and we get more depressed by the year.*

Sensory and Skin Sensitivity

People with CFS and fibromyalgia describe a feeling of sensory overload, a claustrophobic-like feeling that they need to leave a crowded room or location immediately. There can also be a particular skin sensitivity to sounds, and to touch, a feeling that hair bands, eyeglasses, or jewelry can cause sensitivity or pain. These symptoms can extend to very sensitive, tender skin (known as allodynia), or a feeling of burning feet, especially at night.

One particularly unusual symptom is electromagnetic sensitivity, a feeling like you are particularly sensitive to electrical fields. For example, thunderstorms make you feel on edge and uncomfortable. (Note: Some people even report that clocks, watches, and computers stop around them—a form of electromagnetic sensitivity).

Evelyn, a nurse before her fibromyalgia was diagnosed, describes the claustrophobic-like feeling around people:

Being with other people, especially in groups, being in loud, noisy places where there is a lot of activity, make my symptoms much worse. Accepting that has been very difficult for me, especially when my family cannot accept it. But over time, even though I sometimes feel lonely and isolated, I have come to appreciate solitude and silence. The greatest reliefs to me are those days when there is no television, no radio, and even no music, which I love. Alone, and in quiet long enough, my mental confusion clears; problems with concentration and memory and finding the right words go away; the mind-fog clears up and my vision improves. Then I can think, and read, and write, and do needlework and paint . . . and even garden, when my joints allow, all of which give me pleasure.

Clara describes her sensitivity to noise.

Sensitivity to noise (or hyper acuity in medical jargon) is another phenomenon that really has to be experience[d] to be believed. All noises caused a surge of acidic like discomfort in my brain. Not just the obvious jet planes and next door's hammering, but to this day, the gush of a tap or polite applause still causes a wincing pain through my skull, a kind of low grade electric shock sensation. I am among the masses of ME-ers who can't leave the house without earplugs.

Numbness/Tingling

Numbness and/or tingling sensations (known as paresthesia) are common symptoms, especially in the arms and legs. Some people also notice numbness in the hands, especially in the morning.

Jane's major problem since being diagnosed with fibromyalgia is that as soon as she sits, her arms and legs go numb:

I have to stand at meetings, doctors' waiting rooms, and many other places. I can no longer go on trips, because I cannot sit long enough. Just driving across town is torture. The pain and fatigue are nothing compared to these symptoms. I quit going to movies, because I have to stand most of the time in the back.

Melissa's CFS has caused her problems with paresthesia:

It started when I woke up one morning with a pins and needles sensation in my left arm. I thought I had just slept on it wrong, so I continued to get ready for work. After a couple of hours, the pain was still there. The next day, my doctor checked my arm. He said that the skin temperature was lower than it should be and the color had a mottled-effect but the blood flow was at normal levels. He asked me if I leaned on my elbows a lot. I always had, ever since I was little, so I said yes. He said that I had probably wedged the nerve into the bone. He had me go to see a rheumatologist. The answer sounded pretty lame to me, but I knew nothing about medicine. The rheumatologist said I had a form of tennis elbow and sent me for a nerve conduction test. A nerve conduction test is when they hook electrodes to the surface of the skin and below the skin to monitor electrical impulses. I got through the skin portion of the test on both arms but couldn't complete the below the skin part because it was just too painful. They did the test on both arms for a comparison. The results were inconclusive, but I wasn't told that then. My doctor and the rheumatologist told me not to worry about it and to stop leaning on my elbows. In the year that followed, the pain had spread from my left arm to my right arm as well. I was also starting to have pain in both of my legs and other parts of my body as well.

Temperature Sensitivity

A particular reactiveness to temperature changes is another particular type of sensitivity seen in CFS and fibromyalgia. This includes being sensitive to changes in weather, to cold and hot, and to humidity. In particular, some people are susceptible to cold in their hands. For example, the hands hurt, they get pins and needles, or they turn blue when under cold water or exposed to cold, a symptom referred to as Raynaud's phenomenon.

Allergies and Product Sensitivities

Many CFS and fibromyalgia patients complain of sensitivities to chemicals or other substances, allergies, and an intolerance or over-reactiveness to medicines and alcohol. Symptoms can include fatigue, swelling, tearing eyes, rashes, breathing disturbances, bloating, headaches when in contact with various chemicals—everything from cleaning products to gasoline, to pesticides, to solvents—or various pollens, foods, and molds. Regarding medicines, some people need only a small amount of a drug or overreact to a normal-size dose. And even a normal intake of alcohol can cause extreme fatigue in people with these types of sensitivities.

Didi describes her range of allergy and sensitivity symptoms:

. . . I developed a range of symptoms including urticaria (hives), breathing difficulties, strong persistent headaches, also facial mouth, tongue, and airway swelling, sometimes to

the point of total restriction. At this time I began experiencing Multiple Chemical Sensitivity with severe reactions to a wide range of common foodstuffs, and when exposed to gasoline, thinners, methylated and/or white spirits, bleach, household cleaners, and pesticides. These reactions include immediate violent headaches, nausea, dizziness, numbness of face and extremities, swelling of lips and tongue. . . .

Claire found herself dealing with sensitivity to medicines:

I have been mostly fortunate because I have a doc and a therapist who know this disease. They both understand my sensitivity to meds . . . that I can only take miniscule amounts of anything. I have settled on Celexa [about a mg a day], Bextra for pain and 10 mg of a thyroid medication. Other drugs like Wellbutrin landed me in the hospital. Sleep meds have a paradoxical effect on me so despite insomnia, restless leg syndrome and upregulation all being problems for me, I have to find other ways to cope.

Eyes/Vision

Eyes and vision can be affected by CFS and fibromyalgia. Frequently, people will be sensitive to bright or fluorescent lights, or particularly sensitive to oncoming headlights at night. Eyes may be dry, irritated, scratchy, and painful, and vision blurry. Prescriptions frequently change, and other more serious problems such as tunnel vision, floaters, even blind spots may occur.

Mouth/Teeth/Face/Jaws

The mouth, teeth, face, and jaws are common areas for symptoms in fibromyalgia and CFS. Dry mouth, which can lead to more frequent cavities and gum disease, can be a symptom. One more common symptom is aching jaws, particularly in the morning, due to grinding the teeth during sleep and the resulting temporomandibular joint dysfunction (TMD). TMD can also cause jaw and face pain, a clicking or locked jaw, and pain in the temples.

Elimination

One of the more common fibromyalgia and CFS symptoms is irritable bowel syndrome, which typically involves alternating diarrhea and constipation, with bloating and cramping. Urination can also be a problem, with irritable bladder or interstitial cystitis symptoms such as urinary urgency, feeling like you always have to urinate, feeling as if you cannot empty your bladder entirely, or burning and pain during urination.

Digestion

Nausea, indigestion, heartburn, gastroesophageal reflux disease (GERD), and gas are all symptoms that can be seen in CFS and fibromyalgia.

Low Blood Sugar/Hypoglycemia

A fair percentage of people with CFS and, in particular, fibromyalgia experience hypoglycemia, or low blood sugar. It's so common in fibromyalgia that practitioner and founder of the guaifenesin protocol, R. Paul St. Amand, M.D., has coined the term "fibroglycemia."

Dizziness/Balance

Problems with dizziness and balance are fairly common symptoms of CFS and fibromyalgia—in particular, a condition known as "orthostatic intolerance." The theory behind orthostatic intolerance is that there is diminished blood volume or dehydration. Blood therefore pools in the extremities, and the heart's effort to pump and recirculate the blood causes dizziness when a person stands up or gets out of bed. Symptoms include light-headedness, dizziness, fatigue, and fainting. Orthostatic intolerance is one in a number of problems that can affect the autonomic system, and is known as a dysautonomia. Other symptoms that fall into this category include postural tachycardia, where your heart rate rises substantially when you stand or get out of bed, and neurally mediated hypotension, where your blood pressure falls when you stand or get out of bed, and postural hypertension, where your blood pressure rises when you stand or get out of bed. Some people have mild to serious vertigo, a spinning or moving sensation when you are not moving. Fainting and clumsiness are also seen in CFS and fibromyalgia.

Jeri describes her problems with dysautonomia.

Some have orthostatic hypotension, some have neurally mediated hypotension. I have both. My blood pressure sometimes drops below 90/60; if it is around 80/50 I feel more sluggish, lethargic, and sometimes weak.

Vital Signs

The vital signs—blood pressure and body temperature—can be very symptomatic in CFS and fibromyalgia. Low blood pressure, particularly when standing up or getting out of bed, is one more common symptom. Some people have a body temperature gone haywire—very low in the morning, rising to low-grade fever in the afternoon. Others have a chronic low-grade fever, or a temperature that always runs below normal.

Kerrie describes her body temperature issues:

I can see how this has affected me—my temperature tends to go down when I get sick. Recently I had a virus and my temp went to 101, and I panicked. My temp hasn't been that high since I got sick in 1967!

Hair, Skin, Nails

Some CFS and fibromyalgia patients report hair loss as a symptom. Skin can be pallid, or red and mottled in some people. Rashes, itching, dryness and frequent breakouts, scarring and bruising can be more common. Nails are more likely to have ridges, to curve, to be dry and easily broken, with fragile cuticles.

Hormonal/Female Specific

One of the more common CFS and fibromyalgia symptoms is development of premenstrual syndrome (PMS) or worsening of PMS. Symptoms include bloating, weight gain, lower back pain, skin breakouts, tender breasts, sore throat, joint aches and pain, swollen ankles, difficulty sleeping, carbohydrate cravings, anxiety, irritability, fatigue, mood changes, depression. Some women also report painful menstrual periods (known as dysmenorrhea), and pain (known as vulvodynia) in the vaginal area that is not associated with infection.

Sexual/Reproductive Concerns

A reduced or absent sex drive may be seen in some people with CFS or fibromyalgia. Others report impotence or painful intercourse.

Swelling

Some CFS and fibromyalgia patients report swelling (known as edema), or a swollen feeling, most often in the legs, ankles, hands, fingers, or wrists. A particular symptom reported by some CFS and fibromyalgia patients is a swollen feeling in the abdomen or side.

Heart/Cardiac

Some CFS and fibromyalgia patients report experiencing heart palpitations, skipped heartbeats, sensations of thumping or fluttering heartbeat, or have been diagnosed with mitral valve prolapse or other unusual heart rhythms and arrhythmias. A rapid, racing heartbeat (known as tachycardia) is also connected. Some CFS and fibromyalgia patients report having noncardiac chest wall pains or lower rib cage pain, sometimes known as costochondritis.

Immune System/Resistance

People with CFS and fibromyalgia may show signs of lowered immunity, such as more frequent or difficult-to-treat infections, especially sinus infections, ear infections, urinary tract infections, and shingles.

Ellie describes this symptom:

I go through times when I feel like I have absolutely no resistance to every germ in my path. I catch everything, and I mean every single thing, that is going around.

Ears/Hearing

Some people report pain or itching in the ears. CFS and fibromyalgia are also associated with ringing in the ears—known as tinnitus—and frequent ear infections.

Weight/Appetite/Thirst

Weight gain or weight loss that is not associated with a change in eating habits has been linked to CFS and fibromyalgia. In particular, loss or decrease in appetite, increase in thirst, and cravings for carbohydrates, especially sweets, are known symptoms.

Insects and Bites

Some people with CFS or fibromyalgia feel that they attract mosquitoes or flies more than others around them. It's also been reported anecdotally that people with CFS and fibromyalgia have more swelling, hardness, and scarring after an insect bite.

Risk Factors and Symptoms Checklist

God provides the wind,
but man must raise the sails.
—ST. AUGUSTINE

The following risk factor and symptom checklist can help you get diagnosed or serve as a tool for you to work with your practitioner to treat your symptoms better.

■ Risk Factors/Markers

___ Female gender
___ A family history of CFS or fibromyalgia
___ Having a family or personal history of other conditions, including
   ___ Irritable bowel syndrome
   ___ Endometriosis
   ___ Thyroid disease—hypothyroidism, hyperthyroidism
   ___ Mood disorder

___ Chronic or persistent nasal symptoms/sinusitis/sinus infections

___ Ear infections (particularly with CFS)

___ Hysterectomy (particularly with CFS)

___ Miscarriage

___ Irregular menstrual cycle

___ Ovarian cysts

___ Mononucleosis/glandular fever

___ Epstein-Barr virus

___ Having had a recent infection

___ Mononucleosis/glandular fever

___ Epstein-Barr virus

___ Viral meningitis

___ Viral hepatitis

___ Herpes

___ Enteroviruses

___ Hepatitis

___ Salmonella

___ Toxoplasmosis

___ Influenza

___ Family or personal history of autoimmune disease (check all that apply)

___ Addison's disease

___ Alopecia

___ Ankylosing spondylitis

___ Antiphospholipid syndrome

___ Autoimmune hemolytic anemia

___ Autoimmune hepatitis

___ Autoimmune oophoritis

___ Behcet's disease

___ Bullous pemphigoid
___ Celiac disease
___ Chronic inflammatory demyelinating polyneuropathy
___ Churg-Strauss syndrome
___ Cicatricial pemphigoid
___ Cold agglutinin disease
___ CREST syndrome
___ Crohn's disease
___ Diabetes
    ___ Type I diabetes
    ___ Type II diabetes
___ Dysautonomia
___ Endometriosis
___ Eosinophilia-myalgia syndrome
___ Essential mixed cryoglobulinemia
___ Graves' disease
___ Guillain-Barré syndrome
___ Hashimoto's thyroiditis
___ Idiopathic pulmonary fibrosis
___ Idiopathic thrombocytopenia purpura (ITP)
___ Inflammatory bowel disease (IBD)
___ Lichen Planus
___ Lupus
___ Ménière's disease
___ Mixed connective tissue disease (MCTD)
___ Multiple sclerosis
___ Myasthenia gravis
___ Pemphigus
___ Pernicious anemia
___ Polyarteritis nodosa
___ Polychondritis
___ Polymyalgia rheumatica
___ Polymyositis and dermatomyositis

___ Primary agammaglobulinemia
___ Primary biliary cirrhosis
___ Psoriasis
___ Raynaud's phenomenon
___ Reiter's syndrome
___ Rheumatic fever
___ Rheumatoid arthritis
___ Sarcoidosis
___ Scleroderma
___ Sjögren's syndrome
___ Spondyloarthropathy
___ Stiff-man syndrome
___ Takayasu arteritis
___ Temporal arteritis/giant cell arteritis
___ Thyroid disease
___ Ulcerative colitis
___ Uveitis
___ Vasculitis
___ Vitiligo

___ Physical injuries/trauma
___ Hypermobile joints
___ Toxic exposures
___ Severe life stress
___ Type A personality
___ Recent immunizations/vaccinations
___ Use of medications/drugs known to have a link to CFS/
fibromyalgia
   ___ Accutane
   ___ Buspar
   ___ Cordarone
   ___ Depo-Provera
   ___ Desyrel

___ Epogen
___ Ergamisol
___ Lariam
___ Lopressor
___ Neupogen
___ NORVASC
___ Parlodel
___ Prinivil
___ Procardia
___ Procrit
___ Prozac
___ Reglan
___ Tenormin
___ Toprol
___ Wellbutrin
___ Xanax
___ Zestril
___ Zoloft

■ Symptoms

CFS Symptoms—Official Criteria
The official criteria for CFS include the following symptoms:

___ Fatigue that is medically unexplained, of new onset, that lasts at least six months, that is not the result of ongoing exertion, that is not substantially relieved by rest, and that causes a substantial reduction in activity levels.

Plus four or more of the following symptoms:

___ Substantially impaired memory/concentration

___ Sore throat

___ Tender neck or armpit lymph nodes

___ Muscle pain

___ Headaches of a new type, pattern, or severity

___ Unrefreshing sleep

___ Relapse of symptoms after exercise (also known as postexertional malaise) that lasts more than 24 hours

___ Pain in multiple joints without joint swelling or redness.

Fibromyalgia Symptoms—Official Criteria

The official American College of Rheumatology criteria for fibromyalgia include

___ Widespread pain for at least three months. Pain should be on both the left side of the body and the right side, and both above and below the waist. Cervical spine, anterior chest, thoracic spine, or low back pain must also be present.

Plus pain in at least eleven of eighteen specific tender point sites, which include

___ The area where the neck muscles attach to the base of the skull, left and right sides (occiput)

___ Midway between neck and shoulder, left and right sides (trapezius)

___ Muscles over left and right upper inner shoulder blade, left and right sides (supraspinatus)

___ Two centimeters below side bone at elbow of left and right arms (lateral epicondyle)

___ Left and right upper outer buttocks (gluteal)

___ Left and right hip bones (greater trochanter)

___ Just above left and right knees on inside
___ Lower neck in front, left and right sides (low cervical)
___ Edge of upper breastbone, left and right sides (second rib)

PAIN, ACHES, STIFFNESS

___ General muscle pain/myalgias
___ General joint pain/arthralgias
___ General joint stiffness (esp. elbows, knees, hips)
___ Joint stiffness in the morning
___ Joint stiffness after maintaining same position for a length of time
___ Burning or soreness in muscles that becomes worse after exercise
___ Burning or soreness in muscles that worsens later in the day
___ Aching/pain in the upper back and its muscles
___ Aching/pain in the lower back and its muscles
___ Aching/pain in the buttocks
___ Aching/pain in the midback and its muscles
___ Aching/pain in the neck and shoulders
___ Aching/pain when you wear heavy clothing or carry a shoulder bag
___ Moving pain
___ Abdominal pain
___ Aching/pain in the ribs/rib cage area (costochondritis)
___ Breast pain and/or extra-sensitive nipples
___ Aching/pain in the pelvis
___ Aching/pain in the hip that radiates down the leg
___ Sciatica-like pain
___ Aching/pain in the coccyx/tailbone and rectal area
___ Pain in the vaginal area (vulvodynia)
___ Pains or cramps when you write or type
___ Carpal tunnel syndrome–like pains
___ Weak, painful grasp that makes it difficult to hold things

___ Growing pains or chronic aches as a child
___ Painful menstrual periods

MUSCLES
___ Muscle cramps
___ Muscle twitching
___ Muscle spasms

HEADACHES
___ Recurrent tension headaches
___ Recurrent migraine headaches

FATIGUE
___ General tiredness
___ Fatigue alternating with periods of normalcy
___ Extreme exhaustion
___ Fatigue that is not relieved by rest
___ Flulike total body fatigue that does not go away
___ Exhaustion during and after physical and mental stress

EXERCISE AND EXERTION INTOLERANCE
___ Muscle pain, fatigue, and exhaustion after exercise
___ Prolonged fatigue after exercise, lasting twenty-four hours or more
___ Delayed reaction postexertional fatigue
___ Relapse of symptoms after exercise (postexertional malaise)

SLEEP DISTURBANCES
___ Morning fog
___ Sleep apnea—snoring, periodic stopped breathing episodes
___ Sleep myoclonus—nighttime jerking, jumping, and spasming of arms and legs
___ Restless leg syndrome

___ Unrefreshing sleep
___ Frequent waking during sleep
___ Trouble falling back to sleep after awakening during the night
___ Insomnia—trouble falling asleep
___ Nightmares—often unusual and recurring
___ Night sweats
___ A sensation while falling asleep that you have fallen or dropped from a height
___ Frequent nighttime urination (nocturia)
___ Early waking

BREATHING/RESPIRATORY/NOSE/THROAT

___ Shallow breathing
___ Feeling like you can't take a full breath
___ Feeling as if you need to yawn to get a full breath
___ Shortness of breath
___ Hyperventilation
___ Sinus problems
___ Nighttime stuffiness
___ Frequent runny nose
___ Thick nasal congestion that is difficult to clean
___ Regular cough—especially a dry cough
___ Trouble swallowing
___ "Lump in your throat" feeling
___ Sore throat (known as pharyngitis)

COGNITIVE/THINKING/MEMORY/CONCENTRATION

___ Brain fog—general difficulty concentrating
___ Impaired attention span
___ Difficulty or inability to learn new information or skills
___ Poor memory

___ Short-term memory problems, such as inability to remember what you went to the store to buy

___ Feeling easily distracted

___ Problems remembering words or names (verbal memory)

___ Problems remembering things you've seen (visual memory)

___ Slowed reaction time to questions

___ Difficulty absorbing complex information you hear

___ Confusion, difficulty remembering familiar faces, locations, or directions

___ Word confusion, word substitution, difficulty finding the right word

___ Reversing word order or first letter and sounds (known as pseudodyslexia)

___ Problems with numbers and math, from performing equations, to remembering familiar numbers

MOOD/DEPRESSION

___ Feelings of worthlessness, fatigue, and the blues

___ Anxiety, having days when everything makes you nervous, anxious, or irritable

___ Mood swings

___ Noticeable seasonal blues, seasonal affective disorder—SAD

___ Panic attacks—including racing heartbeat, dizziness, feeling of doom

___ Tendency to cry easily

SENSORY AND SKIN SENSITIVITY

___ Sensory overload, a claustrophobic-like feeling

___ Sensitivity to touch

___ Tender skin (known as allodynia)

___ Sensation of burning feet, especially at night

___ Electromagnetic sensitivity

NUMBNESS/TINGLING
___ Numbness or tingling sensations (known as paresthesia), especially in arms and legs

___ Tingling

___ Hand numbness, especially in the morning

TEMPERATURE SENSITIVITY
___ Sensitivity to temperature changes

___ Sensitivity to changes in weather

___ Sensitivity to changes in humidity

___ Sensitivity to cold in hands

___ Sensitivity to cold—especially cold drafts or blowing air, which can trigger pain or stiffness

ALLERGIES AND PRODUCT SENSITIVITIES
___ Multiple chemical sensitivities

___ Allergies and/or sensitivities—to pollen, foods, molds

___ Sensitivity to medicines

___ Sensitivity or intolerance to alcohol

EYES/VISION
___ Waking up with eyes crusted over

___ Sensitivity to lights and brightness

___ Sensitivity to fluorescent lights

___ Night blindness, difficulty driving at night, sensitivity to oncoming headlights

___ Dry eyes

___ Scratchy, irritated eyes

___ Double vision

___ Watery eyes

___ Eye pain

___ Visual blurring or changes

___ Frequent eyeglass or contact lens prescription changes

___ Words jumping or blurring on the page
___ Brief duration patches of blindness
___ Floaters and cloudy spots in vision
___ Tunnel vision
___ Loss of your visual depth of field

MOUTH/TEETH/FACE/JAWS
___ Dry mouth
___ More frequent cavities
___ Gum disease
___ Crimson crescents in the back of the mouth
___ Jaw clenching
___ Jaws aching, especially in the morning
___ Bruxism (teeth grinding)
___ Diagnosis of temporomandibular joint dysfunction syndrome (TMJ, TMD)
___ Jaw and face pain
___ Clicking jaw
___ Jaw that becomes locked or stuck
___ Pain in temples, over jaw area
___ Toothaches unexplained by dental problems
___ More frequent canker sores
___ Prickling, tingling, painful sensation along the jawline that can move upward across the cheeks

ELIMINATION
___ Irritable bladder or interstitial cystitis symptoms
___ Urinary urgency
___ Feeling as if you cannot empty your bladder entirely
___ Burning on urination
___ Pain on urination
___ Diarrhea
___ Constipation

___ Diarrhea and constipation alternating
___ Bloating and cramping
___ Diagnosis of "irritable bowel syndrome"

DIGESTION

___ Nausea
___ Indigestion
___ Heartburn or gastroesophageal reflux disease (GERD)
___ Stomach ulcers
___ Reactive hypoglycemia
___ Gas
___ Hypoglycemia, low blood sugar, "fibroglycemia"

DIZZINESS/BALANCE

___ Dizziness
___ Panic attacks
___ Orthostatic intolerance
___ Heart rate rises substantially when you stand or get out of bed (known as postural tachycardia)
___ Dizziness on rising or moving
___ Dizziness, vertigo (spinning or moving sensation when you are not moving)
___ Dizziness triggered by patterns in floors or light/dark patterns
___ Clumsiness, bumping into things
___ Dropping things
___ Spatial disorientation, difficulty judging distance
___ Spilling food or drink while eating
___ Feeling like your depth perception is off-kilter
___ Fainting

VITAL SIGNS

___ Low blood pressure

___ Low blood pressure when you stand up or get out of bed (postural hypotension)

___ Haywire body temperature—very low in the morning, rising to low-grade fever in the afternoon

___ Recurrent low-grade fever

___ Chronically low body temperature—as one or more degrees below normal

HAIR, SKIN, NAILS

___ Hair loss

___ Pale, pallid, colorless skin tone

___ Skin redness, mottling

___ Frequent rashes

___ Dry, peeling, or itching skin

___ Acne, frequent breakouts

___ Skin that scars easily

___ More frequent bruising

___ Bruises taking longer to heal or fade

___ Ridges in the fingernails

___ Nails that curve under

___ Dry nails that easily break

___ Fragile cuticles that easily tear

___ Cuticles that bleed easily

HORMONAL/FEMALE SPECIFIC

___ Worsened or new premenstrual syndrome (PMS)

___ Fibrocystic breasts

___ Painful menstrual periods (dysmenorrhea)

___ Pain in the vaginal area (vulvodynia)

SEXUAL/REPRODUCTIVE CONCERNS
___ Decreased sex drive/low libido
___ Impotence
___ Painful intercourse
___ Painful menstrual periods

SWELLING
___ Swelling (edema) or swollen feeling in the legs, ankles, hands, fingers, or wrists
___ Swollen feeling in abdomen or side

HEART/CARDIAC
___ Heart palpitations, skipped heartbeats, sensation of thumping or fluttering heartbeat
___ Rapid, racing heartbeat (tachycardia)
___ Diagnosis of mitral value prolapse
___ Unusual heart rhythms, arrhythmias
___ Noncardiac chest wall pains
___ Lower rib cage pain

IMMUNE SYSTEM/RESISTANCE
___ More frequent infections
___ Recurring infections or infections that are hard to treat
___ Periods when your resistance is low and you feel like you are catching everything that is going around

EARS/HEARING
___ Sharp pain in ears
___ Itching in ears
___ Ringing in the ears (tinnitus)
___ Frequent ear infections

WEIGHT/APPETITE/THIRST

___ Weight changes—gain or loss not associated with change in eating habits

___ Anorexia—loss of appetite

___ Decreased appetite

___ Increased thirst

___ Carbohydrate cravings—especially sweets

INSECTS AND BITES

___ Attracting mosquitoes or flies more than others

___ Insect bites becoming more swollen and hard than in others and can leave scars

Getting Diagnosed

Take a cruise, Dorothy.
See a hypnotist.
Change your hair color.
—DOCTOR to Dorothy Zbornak,
Bea Arthur's character on the
sitcom *Golden Girls*, as she sought
a diagnosis for her CFS symptoms

Getting diagnosed as quickly as possible is important, in part because the earlier you are diagnosed, the earlier you can start treatments that may alleviate your symptoms. Some chronic fatigue syndrome (CFS) and fibromyalgia experts believe that your greatest chance of effective treatment—or even cure—exists earlier in the course of the condition. You have tremendous incentive, therefore, to seek a diagnosis as quickly as you can.

Diagnosis of CFS and fibromyalgia can, however, be a difficult and lengthy process. The symptoms can sometimes develop slowly over time, making it harder to put together a clinical picture of CFS or fibromyalgia. The symptoms can also be so similar to other conditions that misdiagnosis is common. And finally, some physicians are either not skilled at recognizing and diagnosing the conditions

or do not acknowledge their very existence, making diagnosis difficult, if not nearly impossible.

■ Seeing the Right Practitioner

Getting a correct diagnosis of your chronic fatigue syndrome or
fibromyalgia assumes that you are seeing the right practitioner. In
order to successfully be diagnosed, you need

- A practitioner who acknowledges the existence of CFS and
  fibromyalgia
- A practitioner who believes you and takes your symptoms
  seriously
- A practitioner who can proficiently diagnose CFS and/or
  fibromyalgia, or who recognizes when it's time to refer you to
  another expert for further evaluation

As you can see, successful diagnosis starts with the right practitioner. That is why I've dedicated chapter 14 to the topic of how to
find and work with the best doctors and practitioners for your CFS
and fibromyalgia diagnosis and care.

You can be as prepared and organized as possible, but if you're
dealing with a closed-minded or uninformed practitioner, you may
be wasting precious time fighting against an insurmountable obsta-
cle to diagnosis.

Angela describes her experience with such a doctor:

*The last doctor that I went to before getting diagnosed with
fibromyalgia said, "All you need is to get married, and have
sex!" Seriously. I left there nearly in hysterics. I was beginning to think that I was crazy, that I was just having mental*

*or emotional problems. Then, I heard about a pain manage-
ment specialist who specialized in fibromyalgia. I went to
him, and he spent almost 2 hours with me, and I just cried
and cried. Finally, someone who knew what was wrong with
me!!*

As an empowered patient, you may feel that it's your job to
reeducate your doctor, or change his or her mind. But do you
have the time and energy to dedicate to your practitioner's continuing education? If you are going to invest time to convince
your doctor of your condition (or even argue for the existence of
CFS and fibromyalgia in the first place), followed by educating
him or her regarding symptoms and treatments, you are delaying your ability to obtain diagnosis and treatment, and potentially delaying your possible recuperation. So think carefully
and decide whether your relationship with this doctor is so good
that it's worth your time and energy, and ultimately worth a
possible delay in your diagnosis or delay in recuperation. If you
can't justify this investment in your physician, then move on
and find a better, more knowledgeable practitioner who already
has a good track record working with CFS and fibromyalgia
patients.

■ Evaluation of Your Full Clinical History

One of the first steps to undertake with your practitioner is an evaluation of your medical history. Go to your appointment prepared
to provide detailed information on the following health history
issues:

- Significant health problems in your parents, siblings, children,
  and other family members

The CFS Evaluation and Diagnosis Process—Conventional

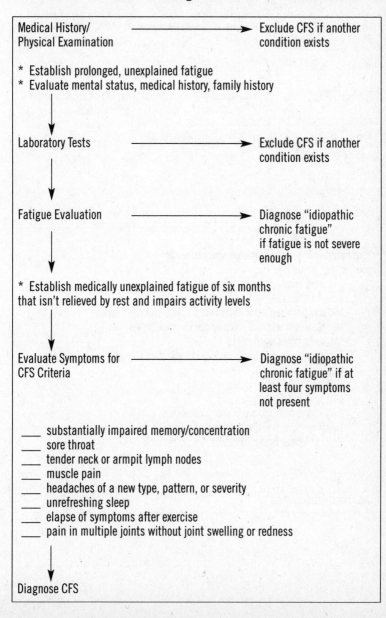

Medical History/
Physical Examination   ⟶   Exclude CFS if another condition exists

* Establish prolonged, unexplained fatigue
* Evaluate mental status, medical history, family history

Laboratory Tests   ⟶   Exclude CFS if another condition exists

Fatigue Evaluation   ⟶   Diagnose "idiopathic chronic fatigue" if fatigue is not severe enough

* Establish medically unexplained fatigue of six months that isn't relieved by rest and impairs activity levels

Evaluate Symptoms for   ⟶   Diagnose "idiopathic
CFS Criteria   chronic fatigue" if at least four symptoms not present

____ substantially impaired memory/concentration
____ sore throat
____ tender neck or armpit lymph nodes
____ muscle pain
____ headaches of a new type, pattern, or severity
____ unrefreshing sleep
____ elapse of symptoms after exercise
____ pain in multiple joints without joint swelling or redness

Diagnose CFS

The Fibromyalgia Evaluation and Diagnosis Process—Conventional

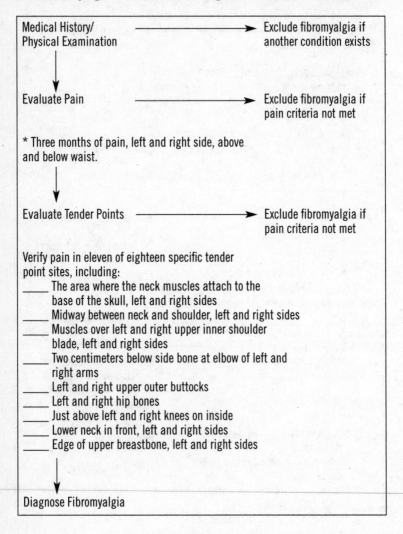

Medical History/
Physical Examination ──────────────► Exclude fibromyalgia if
                                       another condition exists

Evaluate Pain ──────────────► Exclude fibromyalgia if
                               pain criteria not met

* Three months of pain, left and right side, above
and below waist.

Evaluate Tender Points ──────────────► Exclude fibromyalgia if
                                        pain criteria not met

Verify pain in eleven of eighteen specific tender
point sites, including:
_____ The area where the neck muscles attach to the
      base of the skull, left and right sides
_____ Midway between neck and shoulder, left and right sides
_____ Muscles over left and right upper inner shoulder
      blade, left and right sides
_____ Two centimeters below side bone at elbow of left and
      right arms
_____ Left and right upper outer buttocks
_____ Left and right hip bones
_____ Just above left and right knees on inside
_____ Lower neck in front, left and right sides
_____ Edge of upper breastbone, left and right sides

Diagnose Fibromyalgia

- Diseases and diagnoses, past/present
- Psychiatric and mental health history
- Medications you take
- Allergies
- History of injuries and surgeries
- Foreign travel
- Immunizations
- Tobacco use
- Drug use
- Alcohol use
- Sexual activity and birth control
- Caffeine use
- Diet
- Weight
- Exercise
- For women: pregnancy, childbirth, menstrual, and menopausal history
- Employment and insurance information

A listing of current symptoms will also be part of the examination. The Risks and Symptoms Checklist in chapter 4 will be a help to you and your practitioner in summarizing and organizing your symptoms. It's recommended that you fill it out and bring three copies, one for the doctor in the office, one for you to refer to at whatever medical office or testing facility you visit, and one for your file.

■ Evaluation of Your Fatigue and Pain

The next step is more in-depth evaluation of your fatigue and pain, with an eye toward pinning down whether or not you have CFS and/or fibromyalgia, according to your practitioner.

Fatigue is perhaps the most important symptom common to both CFS and fibromyalgia, and often the starting place for diagnosis.

Some surveys report that as much as 20 percent of the general population suffers from long-term, debilitating fatigue. And many patients complain about pain—both specific and nonspecific. Fatigue and pain are two of the most common complaints that bring patients in to see a doctor.

You'll need to be very specific about your fatigue in order to have it taken seriously and not just written off. Fatigue is a very serious concern to patients because it can so frequently be debilitating. But doctors do not tend to take it seriously because it is not specific, and fatigue alone doesn't suggest a particular diagnosis.

As for pain, it's another generic symptom—alone it doesn't point to one clear diagnosis, and it's subjective, so it can't easily be measured.

So at minimum, be prepared to quantify your fatigue and pain.

For example, it's not enough to say, "Being tired has totally disrupted my life." You need to quantify, offer numbers, percentages, and hours, to help doctors understand. For example:

I used to be able to sleep 7 hours a night, and function fine in my 40 hour a week full-time job, plus keep up a 3-bedroom house, and care for my husband and 5 year-old child. Now, I am so tired I can only work a half-day, I need to sleep 3–4 hours in the afternoon, and sleep 10 hours a night, and weekends I am nearly bedridden. I do very little around the house and cannot do more than very basic activities at home and work.

Or, you may want to use percentages. For example:

In January, I was feeling great, and functioning at 100% energy. I had the flu in March, and at that point, felt like I was at about 50% energy. Now it's June, and my fatigue is so debilitating, I feel as if I'm functioning at no more than 30% energy.

Or provide specifics regarding activity levels:

Before the onset of this debilitating fatigue, I was going to the gym 3 times a week for an aerobics class, working out in the weight room twice a week, and spending a few hours every Saturday coaching my child's soccer team. Now, walking up a flight of stairs leaves me at an 8 out of 10 in terms of back and leg pain for an hour. I wake up with pain at about a 7 out of 10 on the scale, and I can go no more than 5 minutes at the slowest speed on the treadmill before I peak out at about a 9 on the pain scale, and feel entirely spent and exhausted.

To help your practitioner understand your pain and/or fatigue, you may want to fill out the Pain and Fatigue Daily Diary/Checklist each day for several weeks, so that you can provide specific records for your physician, documenting these particular symptoms.

Pain and Fatigue Daily Diary/Checklist
Date: _____

Where are you experiencing pain today? (Circle the areas that hurt)

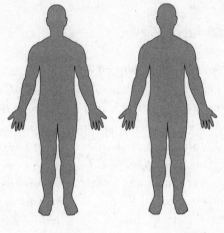

Front   Back

Rate your pain level (morning). My pain is . . .

1	2	3	4	5	6	7	8	9	10

Mild   Uncomfortable/   Excruciating/
                      limits activity   prevents activity

___Aching/soreness   ___Burning/stinging   ___Pins and needles/
                                                    tingling

___Throbbing   ___Steady   ___Sharp

___Dull   ___Constant   ___Starts and stops

Rate your pain level (after exercise). My pain is . . .

1	2	3	4	5	6	7	8	9	10

Mild   Uncomfortable/   Excruciating/
                      limits activity   prevents activity

___Aching/soreness   ___Burning/stinging   ___Pins and needles/
                                                                     tingling

___Throbbing   ___Steady   ___Sharp

___Dull   ___Constant   ___Starts and stops

Rate your pain level (normal daytime). My pain is . . .

1   2   3   4   5   6   7   8   9   10

Mild   Uncomfortable/   Excruciating/
                     limits activity   prevents activity

___Aching/soreness   ___Burning/stinging   ___Pins and needles/
                                                                      tingling

___Throbbing   ___Steady   ___Sharp

___Dull   ___Constant   ___Starts and stops

Rate your pain level (nighttime/in bed). My pain is . . .

1   2   3   4   5   6   7   8   9   10

Mild   Uncomfortable/   Excruciating/
                     limits activity   prevents activity

___Aching/soreness   ___Burning/stinging   ___Pins and needles/
                                                                       tingling

___Throbbing   ___Steady   ___Sharp

___Dull   ___Constant   ___Starts and stops

Rate your fatigue level (morning). My fatigue is . . .

1   2   3   4   5   6   7   8   9   10

Mild   Uncomfortable/   Totally exhausted/
                     limits activity   bedridden

Rate your fatigue level (after exercise). My fatigue is . . .

1   2   3   4   5   6   7   8   9   10

Mild   Uncomfortable/   Totally exhausted/
                     limits activity   bedridden

Rate your fatigue level (normal daytime). My fatigue is . . .

| 1 | 2 | 3 | 4 | 5 | 6 | 7 | 8 | 9 | 10 |

Mild   Uncomfortable/   Totally exhausted/
                         limits activity   bedridden

Rate your fatigue level (nighttime/in bed). My fatigue is . . .

| 1 | 2 | 3 | 4 | 5 | 6 | 7 | 8 | 9 | 10 |

Mild   Uncomfortable/   Totally exhausted/
                         limits activity   bedridden

Other Issues

How many hours were you in bed last night? _____

How many hours of uninterrupted sleep did you get last night? _____

How much and what type of exercise did you do yesterday? _____

How much and what type of exercise did you do today? _____

How many hours of work or school did you miss due to pain today? ____

How many hours of work or school did you miss due to fatigue today? __

Did you smoke today? If so, how many cigarettes? _____

Did you drink alcohol today? If so, how many drinks? _____

Other Notes & Symptoms

_____

_____

_____

_____

_____

Most cases of fatigue are due to factors such as insufficient sleep, general stress, lack of exercise, being overweight, allergies, hormonal imbalances, and other more general causes. And pain most frequently is due to lack of exercise, poor sleep, bad posture, and musculoskeletal misalignment. But in a percentage of cases, fatigue and pain are signs of particular medical conditions. Your physician's taking of medical history, physical examination, and laboratory testing will seek to exclude those conditions that most often cause fatigue or pain, or whose symptoms mimic those of CFS or fibromyalgia.

The conditions your doctor will likely try to rule out include

- Blood disorders, such as anemia (iron deficiency) or lymphoma
- Chronic, undiagnosed infection, such as Lyme disease, chronic hepatitis B and C, HIV, AIDS, tuberculosis
- Autoimmune disease, such as lupus, Sjögren's syndrome, myasthenia gravis or multiple sclerosis, sarcoidosis
- Cancer
- Endocrine problems, such as diabetes, hypothyroidism, or hyper/hypoadrenalism (Addison's or Cushing's disease)
- Sleep disorders such as sleep apnea
- Liver disease
- Heart disease
- Lung disease
- Physical inactivity, lack of exercise
- Allergies, multiple chemical sensitivity
- Musculoskeletal and neurological pain conditions, such as rheumatoid arthritis, polymyalgia rheumatica, sciatica
- Back and neck problems, such as ruptured discs
- Medication side effects (i.e., beta blockers, chemotherapy)
- Heavy-metal toxicity
- Eating disorders (anorexia, bulimia)
- Substance abuse
- Emotional disorders, mental health issues, depression
- Stress—psychological or social
- Anxiety, panic disorder

The CFS Diagnosis Conundrum

One of the most interesting problems with CFS diagnosis is that in addition to the many conditions that share similar symptoms, there are specific conditions that are considered exclusionary factors. Having a past or present diagnosis of any of these conditions prevents a formal diagnosis of CFS being made by a conventional practitioner following the Centers for Disease Control (CDC) guidelines.

These exclusionary factors include, according to CDC guidelines,

Any active medical condition that may explain the presence of chronic fatigue, such as untreated hypothyroidism, sleep apnea and narcolepsy, and iatrogenic conditions such as side effects of medication.

Some diagnosable illnesses may relapse or may not have completely resolved during treatment. If the persistence of such a condition could explain the presence of chronic fatigue, and if it cannot be clearly established that the original condition has completely resolved with treatment, then such patients should not be classified as having CFS. Examples of illnesses that can present such a picture include some types of malignancies and chronic cases of hepatitis B or C virus infection.

Any past or current diagnosis of a major depressive disorder with psychotic or melancholic features:

- *bipolar affective disorders*
- *schizophrenia of any subtype*
- *delusional disorders of any subtype*
- *dementias of any subtype*
- *anorexia nervosa or bulimia nervosa*

Alcohol or other substance abuse, occurring within 2 years of the onset of chronic fatigue and any time afterwards.

Severe obesity as defined by a body mass index [body mass index = weight in kilograms ÷ (height in meters)²] equal to or greater than 45. [Note: body mass index values vary considerably among different age groups and populations. No "normal" or "average" range of values can be suggested in a fashion that is meaningful. The range of 45 or greater was selected because it clearly falls within the range of severe obesity.]

CFS and fibromyalgia expert Dr. Jacob Teitelbaum believes that this list of exclusions ends up actually excluding people who *do* have CFS. One example Dr. Teitelbaum cites is that if someone has at any point been diagnosed with melancholic depression, they can never be formally diagnosed with CFS. Melancholic depression's symptoms can include loss of pleasure/loss of interest in activities that are normally pleasurable, as well as weight loss, brain fog, sleep disturbances, and depressed mood, among others. Since these are also CFS symptoms, having CFS could actually prevent you from being diagnosed with CFS.

Says Dr. Teitelbaum:

Can you imagine if this same exclusion was applied to people with end stage cancer—and that if they fit the very broad criteria for melancholic depression above they would be defined as not having cancer! I would guess that 90 percent of these cancer patients would suddenly technically no longer have cancer (unfortunately they would still die)! What if the implication of this was that they would be denied all health and disability benefits (and research funding) related to the cancer! Sadly, this is what has happened to many people suffering with CFS/fibromyalgia!

According to Dr. Teitelbaum, while almost 12 percent of the population currently has severe disabling fatigue that has lasted at least one month, the CDC's rigorous CFS criteria end up excluding more than 90 percent of possible CFS patients.

Says Dr. Teitelbaum:

The criteria that are being used by the CDC in their epidemiologic studies would mean that most any teenager who ever broke up with a boyfriend or girlfriend in high school would be excluded from ever having the diagnosis of CFS in their lifetime!

Dr. Teitelbaum takes a more liberal approach to CFS and fibromyalgia diagnosis. If someone generally fits the description of CFS or fibromyalgia, with symptoms including unexplained fatigue, plus any two symptoms from among brain fog, sleep disturbances, diffuse achiness, increased thirst, bowel dysfunction, and/or persistent or recurrent infections or flulike feelings, then he believes a positive diagnosis should be assumed.

Fibromyalgia and metabolism researcher Dr. John Lowe believes that fibromyalgia and chronic fatigue are essentially symptoms of the same underlying problem—hypothyroidism/thyroid hormone resistance. Says Dr. Lowe:

The diagnoses doctors give the patients usually depend on the major symptom. For example, if a patient's major symptom is pain, she's likely to get diagnosed with fibromyalgia. If it's fatigue, she's likely to get the diagnosis of chronic fatigue syndrome. Other major symptoms that can lead to different diagnoses include depression unrelated to life events, menstrual abnormalities, high cholesterol, dry skin and mucous membranes, and the list goes on and on. Most of these patients' symptoms are worsened by the same metabolism-impeding factors that worsen fibromyalgia patients' symptoms. What determines a patient's major symptom is the particular body tissues most sensitive to the set of metabolism-impairing factors impinging on the patient.

■ Standard Exclusionary Tests

There are a number of standard tests that are considered useful in the process of excluding the non-CFS/fibromyalgia causes of fatiguing illness. The tests, which were specifically recommended in the CFS case definition article adopted by the CDC, include the following.

Complete Blood Count (CBC)

In a CBC, the red blood cells (erythrocytes), macrophages, neutrophils, basophils, eosinophils, B lymphocytes, and T lymphocytes, among others, are all evaluated. Any variations in the number or appearance of any of these types of cells can be pointers to various illnesses, so a CBC is one of the most basic first-line tests done in the diagnosis of many conditions, including anemia, leukemia, and other disorders.

Erythrocyte Sedimentation Rate (ESR)

What's known colloquially as the "sed rate" indicates the rate at which red blood cells settle out in a tube. An increased sedimentation rate can be a sign of inflammation somewhere in the body.

Alkaline Phosphatase (ALP)

Alkaline phosphatases are a family of enzymes that are present throughout the body. Elevated ALP levels are associated with liver and bile duct disorders, as well as bone diseases.

Alanine Aminotransferase (ALT)

Elevated levels of this enzyme can be an indication of viral hepatitis and other forms of liver disease.

Total Protein

Elevated total protein, measured in plasma, can show dehydration, which might be attributable to vomiting, diarrhea, Addison's disease, diabetic acidosis, and other conditions.

Albumin

Albumin is a protein found in blood plasma. Reduced albumin may point to a variety of conditions, including liver disease, inflammation, malabsorption syndromes, malnutrition, and renal diseases.

Globulin

Elevated levels of globulins, blood plasma proteins, can indicate cirrhosis of the liver.

Calcium

Increased calcium levels may indicate the presence of malignant disease or hyperparathyroidism. Less commonly, they could reflect extreme hyperthyroidism, too much vitamin D, and other disorders. Reduced calcium levels may reflect vitamin D deficiency, renal disease, magnesium deficiency, and other conditions.

Phosphorus

Increased phosphate levels may point to renal failure, hypoparathyroidism, acromegaly, excessive phosphate intake, and vitamin D intoxication. Substantially decreased phosphate levels may reflect vitamin D deficiency, primary hyperparathyroidism, magnesium deficiency, or diabetic ketoacidosis.

Glucose

Elevated blood glucose levels may be an indication of diabetes.

Blood Urea Nitrogen (BUN)

Various kidney diseases can lead to an increase in the level of ureanitogen in the blood.

Electrolytes

Deviations from normal levels of various minerals in the blood, including sodium, potassium, calcium, magnesium, chloride, bicarbonate, phosphate, sulfate, and lactate, can reflect a wide variety of clinical problems.

Creatinine

Elevated levels of plasma creatinine may indicate impaired kidney function.

HIV Antibody

The presence of HIV antibodies can indicate infection or active AIDS, which can be a cause of fatigue.

Thyroid Stimulating Hormone (TSH)

High-normal or elevated TSH levels may indicate hypothyroidism (an underactive thyroid) and low-normal or below-normal levels may suggest hyperthyroidism (an overactive thyroid).

Urinalysis

Urine is typically examined for a variety of diagnostic indicators, including amylase, bilirubin, creatinine, sugars, g-glutamyl transferase, hemoglobin, lactate dehydrogenase, osmolality, electrolytes, myoglobin, protein, urea, and many more. Elevated amylase levels can indicate pancreatic disease; increased urine bilirubin levels signal liver damage or disease; high serum g-glutamyl transferase suggests obstruction or inflammation of the bile ducts or gall bladder, increased lactate dehydrogenase in urine is associated with lupus, bladder cancer, and kidney cancer, among many other conditions.

■ Specialized Tests and Experimental Markers

Beyond what the CDC and conventional physicians consider the standard tests to help exclude a CFS/fibromyalgia diagnosis, there are a number of tests and test results that are considered by some practitioners to help in confirming a diagnosis, or identifying specific conditions that act as markers for higher risk of CFS or fibromyalgia. The CDC labels these tests experimental, and they are, among some circles, considered controversial.

Magnetic Resonance Imaging

Magnetic resonance imaging (MRI) tests may be of help in diagnosing CFS, since they can detect lesions and hyperintensities in the subcortical white matter of the brain, often in the front lobe, which are thought to be more common in CFS. MRI can also help in ruling out suspected multiple sclerosis, a condition that may be suspected in a CFS patient and needs to be excluded.

Single-Photon Emission Computed Tomography

On single-photon emission computed tomography (SPECT), which assesses blood flow to the brain, patients with CFS show significantly higher levels of defects in the cerebral cortex of the brain when compared to normal subjects. In general, SPECT has shown significantly decreased blood flow in CFS patients. SPECT also tends to pick up on more abnormalities than MRIs.

Positron Emission Tomography

Positron emission tomography (PET) scans can show hypometabolism in the brain stem, which can be a marker for CFS.

Transcranial Magnetic Stimulation

Transcranial magnetic stimulation (TMS) can demonstrate impairment to the motor cortex, a potential marker for CFS, showing that the rate of movement is significantly slower in CFS subjects than in controls.

Tilt Table Tests

In a tilt table test, the patient is strapped to a table that can be tilted at various angles. Typically, pulse and blood pressure are measured before and after the incline of the table is changed. In one study most CFS patients were found to exhibit a marked decrease in blood pressure in the tilt table test. Overall, CFS patients have a higher incidence of various autonomic dysfunctions that can be diagnosed by this test, including orthostatic intolerance and neurally mediated hypotension.

Sleep Studies/Sleep Electroencephalography

A substantial percentage of fibromyalgia and CFS patients have an alpha-EEG anomaly, a deficiency in stage 4 sleep, which is the deepest stage of sleep. This deficiency can be demonstrated via electroencephalography (EEG), which can measure brain waves during sleep. Chronic deficiency in stage 4 sleep can contribute to exhaustion, brain fog, and an increased perception of pain.

Candida Albicans

Some experts suspect candida albicans, or yeast, to be a trigger for CFS and fibromyalgia in a percentage of patients. CFS expert Dr. David Bell has stated that as many as 20 percent of his CFS patients have some history of oral candidiasis. Yeast overgrowth can also be detected in the intestinal system and stools via testing such as the specialized stool testing for yeast that is available from the Great Smokies Diagnostic Labs.

Specialized Blood Tests for Infections

Sensitive polymerase chain reaction (PCR) testing is done to identify a variety of infections. A number of infections—including mycoplasma, chlamydia, human herpes virus 6, and others—are more common in CFS and fibromyalgia patients than in the general public. While experts do not understand the specific relationship, there are definitely infectious markers, and in some cases treatment of infection can help resolve CFS and fibromyalgia symptoms. Some practitioners, therefore, suggest that the following panel of tests is essential for all CFS and fibromyalgia patients:

- Mycoplasma panel, for four mycoplasmas (*M. fermentans, M. pneumoniae, M. hominis, M. penetrans*) by PCR
- *Chlamydia pneumoniae* by PCR
- Brucella species by PCR
- *Borrelia burgdorferi* (Lyme disease) by PCR
- Human herpesvirus 6 (HHV-6) test by PCR
- Cytomegalovirus (CMV) test by PCR
- Epstein-Barr virus (EBV) blood test
- Enteroviruses by PCR. *Enteron* is the Greek word for "intestine," and these viruses enter and infect the system through the gastrointestinal tract, going on to affect the nervous system. Some enteroviruses include polio, viral meningitis, and encephalitis. Some researchers have believed that enterovirus infection may be linked to CFS and therefore suggest blood tests or polymerase chain reaction (PCR) examination of muscle biopsy specimens to detect enterovirus infection.

Hormonal Evaluations

• Comprehensive thyroid evaluation. There are some practitioners who believe that an underactive thyroid may be part of the overall series of systemic malfunctions that trigger CFS and fibromyalgia, and that hypothyroidism may be a marker for fibromyalgia and CFS. A thorough thyroid evaluation—not just the thyroid-stimulating hormone (TSH) test, but T4, T3, Free T4, Free T3, Reverse T3, and the thyroid antibody profile—can provide comprehensive evaluation of the thyroid function and determine whether thyroid treatment may be appropriate apart from or as part of the treatment for CFS and fibromyalgia.

• Cortisol levels. Some CFS and fibromyalgia patients have tested low for free cortisol in the 24-hour urine test, as well as elevated evening cortisol in a saliva cortisol testing. Both of these tests may be recommended by your practitioner to assess cortisol production as a measure of the adrenal involvement. Cortisol, which is produced by the adrenal gland, makes the body less resistant to stress and causes additional fatigue, muscle weakness, and pain, among other symptoms.

• When there is some core underactivity in hypothalamic dysfunction present—which is discussed at greater length in chapter 8 and is thought to play a possible role in CFS and fibromyalgia—a reduced adrenocorticotropic hormone (ACTH) response can be seen, along with a more rapid cortisol response. Endocrine testing can help to determine some of these factors.

• Human growth hormone (HGH). Some researchers have found that as many as a third of all fibromyalgia patients have a deficiency in growth hormone. There are also anecdotal reports from some practitioners that there are HGH deficiencies in some CFS patients.

Brain Chemicals

Some research has found that there are imbalances in two brain chemicals—substance P and serotonin—in people with CFS and fibromyalgia. Substance P launches the pain signal process, and serotonin can reduce the intensity of pain signals. Some studies have found elevated levels of substance P and deficiencies in serotonin in CFS and fibromyalgia patients, resulting in their having higher-than-normal intensity of pain messages, with a reduced ability to lessen those pain signals.

Immunologic Tests

A variety of immunologic tests may be performed to assess various immune system markers, some of which may suggest an increased risk of CFS and fibromyalgia:

- Lymphocyte markers (including CD4+ cell counts) may be increased in patients with CFS and fibromyalgia.
- Natural killer cell number/activity/function may be low.
- Immune complexes may be elevated.
- Cytokine assays. Some researchers suggest that elevated levels of certain cytokines, e.g., interleukin-1 and interleukin-6, are associated with CFS. The differences may not be significant enough to be considered diagnostic markers.
- Cell marker assays: At least one study observed an elevation in the number of T cells expressing activation markers among the most severely ill CFS patients. T cell activation markers normally are increased in number on the surface of T cells during periods when the immune system has been engaged in responding to some infectious disease. That work has not been confirmed, and no such trend has been observed in other studies of CFS patients. As such, no set of immune cell markers has yet been identified that serves as a diagnostic tool for CFS.

New Markers?

The search is always on for new markers that make it easier to identify CFS and fibromyalgia. For example, Belgian researchers have found that the presence of a particular protein known as 2-5A binding protein may be a marker for CFS. The protein was found in 88 percent of CFS patients, versus 38 percent of fibromyalgia patients, and 32 percent of healthy people. The protein is part of the immune system's mechanism to fight against viruses.

Some experts have reported that certain types of retroviruses can be detected in the white blood cells of CFS patients using a technique known as the polymerase chain reaction (PCR.) Further research needs to be done on the retrovirus connection to fatiguing illnesses.

6

The Role of Infections

[T]he whole imposing edifice of modern medicine . . .
is like the celebrated Tower of Pisa—slightly off balance.
—CHARLES, Prince of Wales

Since the earliest days after CFS and fibromyalgia began to
become more known, experts have been proposing various theories that these conditions are the direct—or indirect—result of one
or more viral, bacterial, parasitic, or fungal infections.

There is some controversy over whether CFS or fibromyalgia
have any relationship to infection at all. But while not conclusive,
research continues to suggest some sort of connection. For example, in one study conducted by Dr. Garth Nicolson—an expert on
the relationship between infection and diseases such as CFS,
fibromyalgia, rheumatoid arthritis, and Gulf War syndrome—
chronic infections were found in 71 percent of CFS patients versus
12 percent of healthy control subjects.

While studies like this one underscore some sort of role for infection, there's no agreement as to whether the conditions directly
result from active chronic infection, are triggered by latent, inactive
infections that become reactivated, or are evidence of a resolved

infection that triggers an autoimmune response and later develops into CFS or fibromyalgia.

Because the symptoms are so similar, Epstein-Barr virus (EBV), the virus that causes mononucleosis, was a highly suspect viral culprit early in the study of CFS. After much research, it now seems clear that CFS is not directly caused by EBV or by any single specific infectious disease agent. Studies have failed to find a direct cause–effect linkage between any particular infections and CFS or fibromyalgia. At the same time, while there may not be a causal relationship, there does appear to be a strong likelihood that infections contribute to the CFS and fibromyalgia process and are among various causes that lead to the same end point—in this case, CFS or fibromyalgia.

The theory that infections have a role in CFS and fibromyalgia is based on the understanding that infection puts the immune system into a heightened state as the body attempts to fight off the invader. It's thought that in CFS and fibromyalgia, this fight is ongoing, sometimes low-level and chronic, but gradually draining off the immune system resources. Once the immune system is activated, the body produces cytokines, which are proteins released by the immune system as a response to an injury or allergen. These cytokines tell the immune system to ramp up for defense or calm down. Some cytokines start a chain reaction in the body that leads to inflammation and other allergic responses. Some experts believe that key symptoms of CFS and fibromyalgia are the result of these cytokines, and that the immunological dysfunctions of CFS and fibromyalgia patients cause them to overrespond to bacteria, allergens, toxins and parasites, and fail to mount a sufficient response to viruses, fungal infections, and intracellular bacteria like mycoplasma.

It's important to look at the infections that are potentially linked to CFS and fibromyalgia, and some of the treatments being used to deal with these infections.

■ Viral Infection

Many viruses have been studied as part of research on CFS and fibromyalgia, and are thought to have some connection to the conditions. Study of viral pathways and treatments is one of the more active areas of research on the conditions.

Enteroviruses

Enteroviruses, such as Coxsackie viruses A and B, echovirus, and poliovirus, are part of the common picornavirus family. Enteroviruses can cause a variety of infections and symptoms, including subclinical infections, colds, and polio. These infections may become chronic and latent, and experts believe that this may explain some conditions such as post-polio syndrome, cardiomyopathy, juvenile diabetes, and possibly CFS.

Herpesviruses

Herpesviruses, including Epstein-Barr virus, cytomegalovirus, human herpesvirus types 6 and 7, and herpes simplex virus types 1 and 2, have been linked to CFS since study began on the condition. It's thought, for example, that reactivation of the herpesvirus, such as Epstein-Barr virus, may affect the immune system, ultimately resulting in CFS in some patients. Other studies have shown a higher incidence of CFS after mononucleosis, compared to after ordinary respiratory infections. Some studies suggest that there may be a connection between human herpesvirus-6 (HHV 6) and CFS, with one study showing that a high percentage of CFS patients had low-level HHV infection. Dr. Dharam V. Ablashi, D.V.M., M.S., who has served as president of the American Association of Chronic Fatigue Syndrome and is a well-known researcher in the field, found in one study that 54 percent of the CFS patients he evaluated showed signs of reactivated HHV-6 versus only 8 percent of healthy controls. In another study, done by Dr. Garth Nicolson, active HHV-6 infections were seen in 31 percent of CFS patients, versus 9 percent of control subjects.

Stealth Viruses

A stealth virus is a virus that can evade the immune system and avoid being destroyed by modifying genes that instruct the immune system to target these viruses and pathogens. They essentially can replicate and attack without facing any resistance from the immune system. While these viruses damage cells, they don't typically cause the inflammatory, antiviral response that you'd normally see with other viruses—hence, the stealth designation. These viruses are usually spinoffs of human and animal herpesviruses. Several of the so-called "stealth viruses," including a simian cytomegalovirus, have been cultured from CFS patients. These viruses can damage the mitochondria of cells and create defects in the energy-generating metabolic pathways, which may be damaged in CFS and fibromyalgia.

Retroviruses

Retroviruses are an area where there is definitely no agreement as to potential relationship to CFS and fibromyalgia. Some studies looked into a possible link between retroviruses and CFS, but no conclusive evidence has been found. Studies are still ongoing, but some experts recommend that diagnostic testing for retroviruses be done only in potential CFS patients as a way to exclude other diagnoses.

Other Viruses

Other viruses that have been studied and may be associated with CFS and fibromyalgia include lentiviruses, parvovirus B19, and Borna disease virus (BDV), a virus that is linked to depression and schizophrenia, and was found in as many as 34 percent of Japanese CFS patients in one study. Also studied are the so-called "stomach viruses," including Norwalk-like viruses and rotavirus, among others.

■ Bacterial Infection

Chlamydia

Some experts have proposed a link between chlamydial infection and CFS/fibromyalgia. Chlamydial infection is a sexually transmitted disease, caused by a bacterium called *Chlamydia trachomatis*. Chlamydia is transmitted during oral, vaginal, or anal sexual contact, and is one of the most widespread bacterial sexually transmitted diseases in the United States. Dr. Nicolson's research found chlamydia infections in 8 percent of CFS patients versus only 1 percent of control subjects. Some experts believe chlamydia may also be to blame for other conditions, including coronary artery disease, heart attack, and multiple sclerosis.

Mycoplasma

Mycoplasma such as *M. fermentans*, *M. pneumoniae*, and others show the ability to penetrate blood circulation and infect tissues. While experts such as Dr. Garth Nicolson do not believe that these microorganisms cause CFS, fibromyalgia, or related conditions, they are thought to have a role in causing the disease or symptoms to progress or worsen. Dr. Nicolson's own laboratory results have shown mycoplasmal infections in as many as 60 percent of CFS patients and 70 percent of fibromyalgia patients, compared to less than 10 percent of healthy control subjects. In Dr. Nicolson's study, the majority of CFS and fibromyalgia patients had multiple mycoplasmal infections, but multiple infections were not found in any of the controls. Other studies have shown mycoplasma in 50 to 60 percent of CFS and fibromyalgia patients versus 9 to 15 percent of controls, and a European study found 68.6 percent of CFS and fibromyalgia patients were infected by at least one type of mycoplasma, compared to 5.6 percent in the control sample of healthy individuals. Interestingly, 31.4 percent of mycoplasma-positive CFS patients also had HHV-6.

Brucella

Brucella is a bacterium that causes an infectious disease called brucellosis. Brucella is primarily passed among animals, and people become infected by coming in contact with infected animals or contaminated animal products. Brucellosis is not very common in the United States, but is very common in countries with limited animal disease programs or where there are gaps in public health programs. Areas currently listed as high risk are most Mediterranean countries, South and Central America, Eastern Europe, Asia, Africa, the Caribbean, and the Middle East. Unpasteurized cheeses and milks from these areas are a particularly common cause of brucellosis. In addition to eating or drinking brucella-contaminated foods or beverages, one can contract brucellosis by inhalation and via contact with an open wound. People working in slaughterhouses or meatpacking plants, veterinarians, and hunters also may be at greater risk.

Tick-Borne Bacteria

Dr. Cecile Jadin is a Belgian doctor practicing in South Africa. More than a decade ago, a friend of hers became unable to walk and was diagnosed with CFS. Dr. Jadin suspected rickettsial infection, a tick-borne bacterial infection that causes CFS-like symptoms, but tests were negative. The friend developed acute appendicitis, and after removing the appendix, Dr. Jadin sent a sample to Belgium for rickettsiae testing, which was positive. After a three-week course of antibiotic treatment with tetracycline, the friend had recuperated enough to ride her horse and walk again.

Dr. Jadin speculates that one of the initial identified outbreaks of CFS was actually triggered by undiagnosed rickettsial infections:

CFS and Rickettsial infection present with a similar symptomology. . . . CFS was reported in Incline, Nevada, in 1984 and developed into epidemic proportions. Rocky Mountain Spotted Fever originated from the same place in 1916.

The bacteria rickettsiae are known to cause a variety of tick-borne illnesses, including Rocky Mountain spotted fever and rickettsial infection, while *Borrelia burgdorferi* causes Lyme disease, and *Coxiella burnetii* is the cause of Q fever.

Food-Borne Bacteria

CFS and fibromyalgia have been linked to a variety of food-borne bacteria. Some patients report onset of their symptoms and condition after a particular virulent bout with food poisoning. Some of the food-borne bacteria implicated include *Campylobacter jejuni,* shigella, *E. coli,* salmonella, cholera, *Clostridium botulinum, Yersinia enterocolitica, Listeria monocytogenes,* and toxoplasma. Fish-associated toxins such as ciguatera can cause a variety of neurological symptoms, and may play a role in the development of CFS. For more discussion of ciguatera and other toxic overexposures, see chapter 10.

The most common culprits for infection food-wise include

- Foreign tap water
- Undercooked eggs or egg dishes
- Shellfish, including mussels, oysters, or scallops
- Wild mushrooms
- Undercooked meat or wild game
- Unpasteurized milk, cheese, eggnog, ice cream, or juices
- Home-canned goods

- Food in corroded metal containers
- Fresh produce, including fruit
- Hot dogs and deli meats
- Soft cheeses or cheese sauces

■ Parasitic Infection

A variety of parasites have been implicated as potentially involved in the infectious pathway triggering CFS and fibromyalgia. These include

- Giardia, which causes giardiasis
- *E. histolytica,* which causes amebiasis
- *Cryptosporidium parvum,* which causes cryptosporidiosis
- *Cyclospora cayetanensis,* which causes cyclosporiasis
- *Trichinella spiralis,* which causes trichinosis
- Tapeworms and flatworms, which cause cysticercosis, anisakiasis, and other worm infections

■ Fungal Infections: Chronic Yeast/Candidiasis

Chronic overgrowth of the *Candida albicans* type of yeast—a condition known as candidiasis or candida syndrome—is thought to be another infectious agent in the CFS/fibromyalgia picture. There is some evidence that *Candida albicans* infection depresses the immune system, which may provide a hospitable climate for CFS and fibromyalgia. Some practitioners have found that CFS patients respond to antifungal drugs and a diet to minimize intestinal candidiasis.

■ The Lerner Theory

One practitioner, Dr. A. Martin Lerner, himself a CFS patient, has proposed that CFS is due to a definable viral cause. According to Dr. Lerner, a board-certified internist, there is a group of CFS sufferers who have prolonged, chronic mononucleosis after being infected with Epstein-Barr (EBV), human cytomegalovirus (HCMV), or both, and/or possibly human herpesvirus 6 (HHV-6). Viral infection continues in the heart, causing left ventricular dysfunction, which then produces exercise intolerance. Any exertion then worsens cardiac dysfunction. Some studies do indicate that CFS patients have significantly higher rates of abnormal cardiac readings and a high incidence of left ventricular dysfunction.

■ Conventional Treatments

Even some of the most holistic and naturally oriented practitioners will, when treating some types of infections, turn to prescription drugs, particularly when dealing with difficult viruses.

Viral Infections
- Enteroviruses—antiviral prescription drugs, especially acyclovir (Zovirax), are often prescribed.
- Herpesviruses—the antiviral prescription drugs are typically prescribed. For Epstein-Barr virus, often no drugs are given, but in serious cases, acyclovir (Zovirax), is sometimes used. Cytomegalovirus is treated with ganciclovir (Vitrasert, Cytovene). Human herpesvirus (like genital or oral herpes, or shingles) is treated with acyclovir (Zovirax), famciclovir (FAMVIR), or valacyclovir (VALTREX).
- Stealth viruses—with stealth viruses, the main approach cen-

ters on preventing further spread of the virus, and in some cases, ganciclovir (Vitrasert, Cytovene) has been found effective.

For some viruses, various forms of immunotherapy, such as intravenous immunoglobulin (IVIG), are used as treatment. More information on immunotherapy is provided in chapter 7.

Lerner is a proponent of long-term and sometimes lifelong use of antiviral drugs—such as valacyclovir (VALTREX), ganciclovir (Vitrasert, Cytovene), acyclovir (Zovirax), and famciclovir (FAMVIR)—for CFS treatment. Lerner claims that taking a maintenance level of valacyclovir, he was able to work full-time, exercise and swim regularly, according to the ImmuneSupport.com News Service.

Lerner's diagnosis methodology, patented in 2002, includes a complicated program of testing for EBV and HCMV, various antibodies to EBV and HCMV, followed by treatment with antiviral drugs, and claims to alleviate chronic fatigue syndrome. According to his patent,

> *Based on clinical tests, chronic fatigue syndrome is a persistent herpes virus infection including incomplete virus multiplication and thus administration of antiviral agents is shown to alleviate the symptoms associated with the disorder. Based on therapeutic trials, patients receiving the recommended antiviral treatment have experienced significant reduction or elimination of the symptoms associated with chronic fatigue syndrome.*

Bacterial Infections

Most bacterial infections are treated with antibiotics. Antibiotic therapy is an area of great interest for CFS and fibromyalgia, as some experts theorize that resolving the infections that trigger the immune reactions in the first place may be able to aid in the recovery process.

In one study, follow-up was conducted over three years among members of the Shasta CFIDS Association in Northern California. Among those in the group who tested positive for mycoplasma and went on antibiotic therapy, 80 perccent recovered from 50 percent to 100 percent of their preillness health within a three-year period.

Note: Some patients who begin treatment for infections will experience what's known as a Herxheimer reaction, which is a temporary worsening in symptoms due to die-off or release of the toxins from the damaged microorganisms or parasites. Ultimately, the Herxheimer reaction will resolve, and recovery can begin. Long-term infection usually requires long-term treatment, potentially more than a year.

Chlamydia. The antibiotic of choice for chlamydia is azithromycin (Zithromax), followed by doxycycline (Bio-Tab, Vibramycin, Doryx), ofloxacin (Floxin), and sometimes erythromycin (E.E.S., E-Mycin) or amoxicillin (Trimox, Amoxil)

Mycoplasma. Mycoplasma infection requires long-term antibiotic therapy, usually multiple six-week courses of doxycycline (Bio-Tab, Vibramycin, Doryx), ciprofloxacin (Cipro), azithromycin (Zithromax), or clarithromycin (Biaxin). Some experts believe that six months of continuous antibiotics may be necessary for patients with blood infections.

Brucella. For brucellosis, doxycycline (Bio-Tab, Vibramycin, Doryx) and rifampin (Rimactane, Rifadin) are used in combination for six weeks to prevent infection recurrence.

Rickettsia. Tetracycline antibiotics are mixed with various quinolones, and Macrolides antibiotics, as well as metronidazole (Flagyl).

Lyme disease. Amoxicillin (Trimox, Augmentin), doxycycline (Bio-Tab, Vibramycin, Doryx), cefuroxime axetil (Ceftin), or azithromycin (Zithromax) are typically given.

Q Fever. Tetracyclines, doxycycline (Bio-Tab, Vibramycin, Doryx), and chloramphenicol (Chloromycetin) are prescribed. Quinolone antibiotics include

- Ofloxacin (Floxin)
- Ciprofloxacin (Cipro)
- Levofloxacin (Levaquin)
- Sparfloxacin (Zagam)
- Gatifloxacin (Tequin)
- Moxifloxacin (Avelox)
- Trovafloxacin (Trovan)

Macrolides antibiotics include

- Azithromycin (Zithromax)
- Clarithromycin (Biaxin)
- Clindamycin (Cleocin)
- Erythromycin (E.E.S., Eryc, E-Mycin)
- Lincomycin

Keep in mind that many physicians now recommend that if you are taking antibiotics, whether a short-term or long-term course, you should take a quality brand of probiotics, one that at minimum includes *Lactobacillus acidophilus* and *Bifidobacterium longum*.

Food-Borne Bacteria

Shigella. Trimethoprim-sulfamethoxazole (Septra) or a quinolone antibiotic is indicated

Salmonella. Cephalosporin (Keflex) antibiotic

Escherichia Coli. Quinolone antibiotic or trimethoprim-sulfamethoxazole (Septra)

Yersinia enterocolitica **infection.** Cephalosporin (Keflex) when needed

Parasitic Infections

Giardia. Metronidazole (Flagyl)

Cryptosporidium. Paromomycin (Humatin) for severe cases

Cyclospora cayetanensis. Trimethoprim-sulfamethoxazole (Septra)

Trichinella spiralis, which causes trichinosis. Corticosteroid drugs such as prednisone (Deltasone) or hydrocortisone (Cortef) are given, plus an anthelmintic (antiworm) drug, including mebendazole (Vermox) or thiabendazole (Mintezol), and albendazole (Albenza)

Tapeworms and flatworms, which cause cysticercosis, anisakiasis, and other worm infections—anthelmintics are given, including praziquantel (Biltricide) and albendazole (Albenza), plus corticosteroids and anticonvulsants as needed

Chronic Candidiasis/Yeast Infection

System or local antifungals are prescribed, including

- Fluconazole (Diflucan)
- Ketoconazole (Nizoral)
- Miconazole nitrate (Monistat)
- Nystatin (Mycostatin)
- Clotrimazole (Mycelex, Lotrimin, Femizole-7)

■ Complementary Remedies

While some of the viruses and bacterial infections mentioned really do require antibiotic treatment, there are many for which prescription drugs are not given. Doctors rely on your body's own ability to fight off the infection, or there isn't a particular drug known to have an effect on the condition. In other cases, the user of the antiviral or antibiotic drugs needs to be supported by other complementary approaches that can support the immune system, and help minimize any side effects from these potent medicines.

Natural Antiviral Remedies

While you'll want to consult with your practitioner to develop a comprehensive, integrated program to deal with any underlying infections, some of the most commonly recommended natural antiviral treatments include the following:

Vitamin C. Some experts believe that viruses are particularly susceptible to Vitamin C at high doses (usually to bowel tolerance, just below the point at which the supplement causes loose bowels or diarrhea).

Zinc. Zinc, which is becoming increasingly popular to fight the cold virus, has potent antiviral properties against other viruses as well. Some preliminary research has found that supplementation with zinc can help to restore function in the thymus, a key immune organ.

Digestive enzymes. Digestive enzymes come in three types: proteolytic enzymes, which help digest protein; lipases, which help to digest fat; and amylases, which help to digest carbohydrates. Use of enzymes can aid in proper absorption of food. The theory behind this is that undigested foods are able to pass through the intestinal layer (a phenomenon known as "leaky gut syndrome") and these oversized particles are perceived as allergens or pathogens by the immune system, which mounts an inflammatory attack. The enzymes break down the undigested particles until they are too small to cause a reaction. The proteolytic enzymes are also thought to help improve immune system function as well.

Probiotics. A probiotic is an organism that helps to balance the intestinal tract. Probiotics are also frequently referred to as "friendly" or "good" bacteria. Many people are familiar with acidophilus, one of the most well known probiotics, and the "good bacteria" or "live bacteria" found in most yogurts. When you eat foods containing probiotics or take probiotic supplements, the probiotics help to maintain a healthy intestinal tract, and can actually help prevent some illness, or fight off other illness and disease.

These probiotic bacteria are those that, when present in sufficient quantities in your intestines, will kill off and prevent overgrowth of harmful bacteria—pathogenic bacteria—that can lead to digestive problems and disease. More and more, it's thought that regular use of probiotics may be an important way to modulate the immune system. Again, a quality brand of probiotics, one that at minimum should include *Lactobacillus acidophilus* and *Bifidobacterium longum,* is recommended.

Thymic protein/thymus glandular. The thymus is a gland located under your breastbone. In a newborn, it is similar in size to the heart, continues growing until age two or three, and then stays the same size until puberty, at which point it begins to shrink. By age forty, the thymus is reduced to about one-sixth its original size, and the elderly have almost no thymic function. The thymus is a critical part of the immune system. It is in our thymus gland where cancer- and infection-fighting T cells mature. So a shrinking thymus leaves less space for maturation of T cells, and reduces our immunity and ability to fight off infection. One supplement thought to help is thymic protein. To prepare thymic protein, thymus cells from cows are grown in a laboratory and then purified. (Since it's made of purified cells, and not a whole animal, there's no risk of mad cow disease.) Clinical research is already under way, but anecdotal reports from patients and practitioners point to many positive results. Overall, thymic protein is claimed to

- Strengthen the ability to fight infection
- Fight active infections, such as colds, herpes, shingles, flu, sinusitis

- Help treat chronic viral infections
- Decrease viral loads of viruses such as Epstein-Barr virus and others
- Increase white blood cell count
- Increase T cell levels
- Increase white cell count
- Improve symptoms in chronic fatigue syndrome and fibromyalgia

In a small clinical trial of patients with Epstein-Barr virus, participants took 4 mcg of thymic protein three times daily for sixty days. After treatment, the Epstein-Barr virus levels were reduced in two-thirds of patients, and in one case, the levels dropped by 75 percent. Meanwhile, all of the patients reported feeling generally better, with most reporting greater energy and needing less sleep.

Dr. Jacob Teitelbaum recommends thymic protein for people who have chronic viral syndromes, chronic fatigue syndrome that appears to be viral in origin, or has been exposed to or is fighting off a virus.

Noted natural medicine expert Julian Whitaker, M.D., director of the Whitaker Wellness Institute in Newport Beach, California, has said that thymic protein is "likely the most powerful stimulant of the immune system ever discovered."

Note: I use thymic protein, and have to report that I have had fantastic results. With a preschool child who frequently comes home with various colds and viruses, I am often exposed to them. When I feel like I'm coming down with something, I take two to three packets of thymic protein a day (it's a nearly tasteless powder that you put under your tongue so it can be absorbed sublingually), and I have been able to ward off several colds in progress. I've also given it to my preschooler, and it prevented her colds from developing into full-scale illnesses with resulting ear infections.

There are several brands of thymic protein. The one I take is ProBoost, from Genicel Inc. Each packet has 4 mcg of freeze-dried, purified Protein A from calf thymus cell culture, delivering twelve trillion active molecules.

Vitamin B complex. A variety of B vitamins together help in proper immune function.

Pantothenic acid. Pantothenic acid helps the body obtain energy from carbohydrates, fats, and protein; improves the body's ability to cope with stress; supports adrenal function; and fights infections by helping to build antibodies.

Raw garlic/capsules. Garlic has a long proven history as an effective antibiotic, antiviral, antiparasitic, and antifungal.

Lysine. The supplement lysine is known to have potent effect against various viruses, and the herpesvirus family in particular.

L-cysteine. L-cysteine is an amino acid that is converted in the body to N-acetyl cysteine (NAC), which is a strong antioxidant. L-cysteine also helps support the liver's detoxification function.

Camu-camu fruit powder. According to anthropologist and South American herbal expert Dr. Viana Muller, camu is a potent natural antiviral. Says Dr. Muller:

> A high quality camu-camu fruit powder grown wild in South American rainforests has produced spectacular results with all types of herpes viruses, including Epstein Barr and Herpes Zoster (shingles). I have seen it work much faster than Acyclovir, the standard anti-herpes medication and better than L-lysine, a common holistic treatment.

Natural Antibiotics

Probiotics. The importance of probiotics, which can act as potent natural antibiotics, was discussed under the antiviral section, and cannot be emphasized enough.

Olive leaf extract. The active ingredient in olive leaf extract is oleuropein, a substance that strengthens the olive tree against attacks by insects and bacteria. Oleuropein contains a chemical called elenolic acid, which acts as a natural antibiotic and antiviral, helping to balance bacteria levels and restore immune balance.

Beta-glucan. Beta-glucan is a special kind of polysaccharide derived from the cell walls of baker's yeast. Beta-glucan is a powerful immune system stimulator. Macrophages (a type of cell that serves as the immune system's first line of defense) have special receptors for yeast beta-glucan, so taking beta-glucan can activate the macrophages and help make the immune system more effective.

Herbs. Sage, thyme, oregano, and parsley are all herbs you can add to your food that are considered to have antibiotic and antimicrobial properties.

Raw garlic. Garlic, particularly raw garlic, has shown strong antibiotic properties.

Echinacea. Echinacea is a popular herb, used for centuries in the Native American community as a treatment for colds, flu, and other viral illnesses. Echinacea has specific antiviral and antibacterial properties, and activates the immune system to fight against infection. Echinacea is most effective when taken six to eight weeks, then several weeks off before starting again, so the herb does not lose its potency.

Goldenseal. Goldenseal is considered a strong antifungal and antibacterial, and a complement to echinacea. Many supplements actually package the two herbs together. Goldenseal has been a popular herbal remedy for upper respiratory infections and fungal infections.

Grapefruit Seed Extract. Grapefruit seed extract is an antimicrobial that can fight against a variety of viruses, bacteria, fungi, and parasites without killing beneficial bacteria in the intestinal tract. It is considered safe for ongoing, long-term use, and has no reported side effects or interactions, except the possibility of reaction in those who are allergic to citrus fruits.

Natural Candidiasis Approaches

For chronic candidiasis, most practitioners recommend that therapy with an antifungal drug be complemented by a number of approaches, including

- Probiotics—again, quite highly recommended as a mainstay in natural approaches to dealing with candidiasis
- Dietary modification to restrict or eliminate sugar, simple carbohydrates, alcohol and fermented beverages, fruit juices, and foods that contain high levels of yeast
- A practitioner-directed detoxification regimen or cleansing diet
- Increased dietary fiber—but not in the form of breads or grains—to 20–45 grams per day in divided doses
- Fresh garlic (several cloves per day)
- Caprylic acid—a supplement that has particular effectiveness against candida

7

The Immune System

People of genius whenever they are faced with
misfortune find resources within themselves.
—BROUHOURS

■ The Immune System

Some experts believe that CFS and fibromyalgia represent a malfunction in the immune system, and there is some evidence to support that theory as one of the pathways by which these conditions
develop. To understand how CFS and fibromyalgia may potentially
be linked to the immune system, it's important to understand how
the system works.

The immune system is the body's defense system, protecting us
against bacteria, pathogens, microorganisms, cancer cells, and
other things that can be hazardous to our health.

The immune system is in particular on the alert for antigens,
which are large molecules (usually proteins) that travel on the surface of cells, viruses, fungi, bacteria, and certain toxins, such as
chemicals and drugs. When your immune system is working properly, it will identify and destroy anything carrying an antigen. Since
our bodies have some cells that are antigens, a properly functioning

immune system also learns to recognize "normal" antigens and not attack them.

The body has a number of mechanisms that act as the front line against antigens. These include the skin, stomach acid (which can neutralize some antigens), mucus (which can trap some antigens, such as inhaled pollen), tonsils, adenoids, coughs, and tears. We also have the thymus gland, the lymph nodes throughout the body, the bone marrow, and various types of white blood cells, which can attack antigens when they are detected.

In many cases the response to an antigen is inflammation. For example, when you inhale a cold virus, your nasal passages become inflamed. The inflammation process causes the body to release chemicals, among them histamine. The swelling also helps isolate the antigen from body tissues and prevents its movement throughout the body. The inflammatory process and chemicals released also attract white blood cells to destroy antigens or damaged cells.

When you get into a discussion of all the different cells that make up the immune system, things get more complicated. The majority of immune system cells are lymphocytes, which are small white blood cells. Lymphocytes move between blood and tissue. The main types of lymphocytes are B cells, T cells, and killer cells.

Some immune cells are myeloid cells—these are large white blood cells that can devour cells and particles. Myeloid cells include eosinophils and basophils. Eosinophils and basophils are mainly involved in allergic responses, and secrete toxic chemicals to destroy antigen/antibody complexes.

Some myeloid cells become phagocytes. Phagocytes are large white cells that can engulf and digest foreign invaders. They include monocytes, which circulate in the blood, and macrophages, which are found in tissues throughout the body. Macrophages are versatile cells; they act as scavengers, secrete a wide variety of powerful chemicals, and play an essential role in activating T cells.

Neutrophils, cells that circulate in the blood but move into tissues where they are needed, are not only phagocytes, but also granulocytes: They contain granules filled with potent chemicals. These chemicals, in addition to destroying microorganisms, play a key role in acute inflammatory reactions. They ward off and treat bacteria and other antigens but die in the process.

T Cells

Going back to lymphocytes, two major types of lymphocytes are B cells and T cells. T cells, which come from the thymus, help to destroy infected cells and coordinate the body's overall immune response. Their purpose is to remember nonself antigens, and when they encounter those substances, to protect the body in various ways.

The T cell has a molecule on its surface called the T-cell receptor. This receptor interacts with molecules called MHC (major histocompatibility complex). Think of the T-cell receptor as a lock and the MHC as a key. The MHC molecules on the surfaces of most other cells are the key that fit into the T cell's "lock" and allow the T cell to recognize antigens.

Some T cells are called "helper cells," and are identified by surface markers. These are known as "special cluster determined," or CD, cells. CD4 T cells are known as "helper cells," and help or promote immune response. CD8 T cells are "suppressor cells," and suppress or block immune response.

The chief tool of T cells are cytokines, which are chemical messengers secreted by the T cells. Cytokines bind to specific receptors on target cells and then recruit other cells to aid in the immune response. Cytokines can encourage cell growth, promote cell activation, direct cellular traffic, and destroy target cells—including cancer cells and viruses. Because they serve as a messenger between white cells, or leukocytes, many cytokines are also known as interleukins.

Tumor necrosis factor (TNF) is a chemical released by

macrophages and activated T cells. TNF can cause fever and even kill some kinds of cancer cells.

B Cells

The other type of lymphocyte, B cells, work by secreting antibodies. Each B cell produces one specific antibody. When a B cell meets its partner antigen, it starts to create plasma, and the plasma then generates the antibody against that antigen.

Killer Cells

There are also types of lymphocytes called killer cells, including cytotoxic T cells and natural killer (NK) cells. Cytotoxic T cells need to recognize a specific antigen in order to act. On the other hand, NK cells roam and act spontaneously, and don't require specific antigens in order to move into action. Both cytotoxic T cells and NK cells bind to their target and deliver chemicals that kill the invading antigens and cells.

NK cells play a key role in fighting cancer, and they also release interferons, which can prevent or slow viral replication.

Antibodies

Antibodies are made to match up with different antigens. What's particularly interesting about antibodies is that they are shaped in such a way as to match up with an antigen—again, the way a key fits into a lock.

Antibodies belong to a family of large protein molecules known as immunoglobulins. Scientists have identified nine different types among five classes of human immunoglobulins: four kinds of IgG and two kinds of IgA plus IgM, IgE, and IgD.

IgG, the major immunoglobulin in the blood, can enter tissue spaces; it works efficiently to coat microorganisms, speeding their uptake by other cells in the immune system. IgD, found in the membrane of B cells, has a role in helping B cells recognize antigens. IgE is normally found in only trace amounts, but it is responsible for allergy symptoms. IgM, produced to fight antigens, functions primarily as a bacteria killer, but decreases and allows IgG to take over. IgA is a major antibody in body fluids and secretions such as tears, saliva, and the gastrointestinal system, and works as a barrier to guard the entrances to the body.

■ Immune Disorders

Sometimes this complicated immune system does not work the way it should. It may have a response that is not appropriate. It may overrespond, or not respond enough, when it encounters an antigen. It may look at an inherently harmless substance, and react as if it is an antigen. This is what happens when someone has an allergy to something that is otherwise safe for most people, such as, for example, apples, or peanuts.

There are immunodeficiency disorders and immune problems such as Acquired Immune Deficiency Syndrome (AIDS). In these dysfunctions, there is a failure in all or part of the immune system. In AIDS, for example, a virus destroys helper T cells, and ends up being propagated in the body by macrophages and other T cells. Sometimes, the immune system can be deliberately suppressed, such as in chemotherapy, or in giving immunosuppressive drugs to transplant patients so they don't reject a transplanted organ.

The key immune dysfunctions related to CFS and fibromyalgia include

- Allergies
- Leaky gut
- Autoimmunity
- Th1/Th2 imbalance

Allergies

Allergies are an immune system malfunction—the body perceives as a danger something that is normally harmless. Allergies to substances such as pollen or peanuts or dog dander occur when the body's first exposure to that substance triggers an inappropriately large antibody response. So, for example, after that first pollen exposure, or after an unusually heavy exposure, B cells make large amounts of pollen antibody, IgE. The IgE attaches to mast cells, cells found in the lungs, skin, tongue, and linings of the nose and gastrointestinal tract. The next time the person encounters pollen, the IgE-primed mast cells release powerful chemicals that cause wheezing, sneezing, and other allergic symptoms.

Autoimmunity

Autoimmunity is a common form of immune dysfunction. The word *auto* is the Greek word for "self." As late as forty years ago, medical experts believed that the immune system could only be directed against foreign invaders, but researchers discovered that the immune system can become confused and attack "self," targeting the cells, tissues, or organs of our own bodies. Misidentifying "self" as a foreign invader, the immune system moves to be rid of the invader, starting with the manufacture of antibodies—known as autoantibodies—and generation of T cells that have as their mission the destruction of the invader.

"Autoimmune disease," therefore, refers to disease in which the attack on your own cells, tissues, and organs produces inflammatory reactions and other symptoms. More than eighty chronic illnesses fit into this category, each very different in nature, and they can affect everything from the endocrine glands—such as the thyroid—to organs such as the kidneys, to the digestive system. An estimated fifty million Americans, 75 percent of them women, suffer from autoimmune diseases in the U.S., according to the American Autoimmune Related Diseases Association.

Autoimmune disease symptoms include everything from fatigue to joint pain to depression, to numb hands and feet, to heart palpitations—all signs that the immune system has turned upon itself, causing autoimmune conditions such as thyroid disease, diabetes, multiple sclerosis, rheumatoid arthritis, psoriasis, and irritable bowel syndrome. Some experts believe that CFS and fibromyalgia are autoimmune conditions, citing that symptom overlap, elevated antibody levels—including antinuclear antibodies, antipolymer antibodies, and antithyroid antibodies among others—immune complexes, and other immune system abnormalities are all evidence of the connection.

It was thought that a key difference between CFS/fibromyalgia and other autoimmune diseases is that there is no associated inflammation or tissue damage typical of autoimmune disease. Recent research, however, has shown that as many as 30 percent of fibromyalgia patients test positive for the presence of cytokines in skin, indicating some sort of neurological inflammation that may be contributing to the pain symptom.

Leaky Gut

One particularly important area of the immune system is in the intestinal lining, or the gut. A substantial number of immune system cells are located in the gut, and the gut's defense capabilities are particularly susceptible to any disruption, such as food allergies, lactose intolerance, gluten sensitivity, and candida/yeast overgrowth. These sorts of conditions make the gut permeable and incapable of mounting an entirely effective immune defense, causing what's referred to as "leaky gut." A leaky gut allows incompletely digested proteins to pass through and enter the bloodstream, where they activate the immune system. This leads to an inflammatory immune response. When the gut is consistently facing disruptive forces, it becomes increasingly permeable, leading to a chronically activated immune system.

Th1/Th2 Cytokine Imbalance

In some CFS patients, the immune system shows evidence of constantly fighting off perceived assault, or what's known as "chronic activation." It's thought that there may be some sort of unidentified continuing infection or autoimmune process in action. While the immune system may be in overdrive, it's not particularly efficient or effective in most CFS patients. T cells and natural killer (NK) cells, which are charged with the job of destroying infected or cancerous cells, are not particularly effective at proliferating or destroying cells.

Some of the future directions for CFS treatment will focus on efforts to shift the T-helper cell response from Th2 to Th1 patterns.

One important research paper presented by Dr. Roberto Patarca-Montero in *The Journal of Chronic Fatigue Syndrome* discusses how people with CFS tend to have poor immune cell function and a predominance of what's known as "T-helper (Th)2-type cytokine response" when their immune system is activated. T-helper type 2 (Th2) cells attack larger antigens by stimulating B cells to produce antibodies. This is called humoral immunity. In CFS more Th2-type cytokine, known as interleukin-5, is produced, and T-helper cells produce less T-helper type 1 (Th1) cytokines, substances that convey messages to other cells and mediate their function. Th1 cells stimulate macrophages and NK cells, which then attack infectious microbes. This is called cellular immunity.

In a Th2-type response, the body produces cytokines such as interleukin (IL)-4,-5, and-10, activating B lymphocytes, which make immunoglobulins. Overproduction of immunoglobulins is also associated with autoimmune disease.

Dr. Patarca-Montero looked at a variety of therapies designed to target the immune system, in particular those treatments that were attempting to change the balance of cytokines, helping to decrease the Th2-type predominance and allowing greater predominance of a Th1-type response.

■ Immunotherapy Treatments

Mycobacterium Vaccae Injections

One treatment that has appeared to be of help in pushing the immune system toward a Th1 response is vaccination using killed *Mycobacterium vaccae*. Some research has shown improvements in symptoms and food allergies from a series of injections over several months.

Staphylococcal Vaccine

One study found that weekly injections of a staphylococcal vaccine generated a Th1-type predominance, providing some improvement in symptoms for a minority of patients. In one double-blind placebo-controlled study, patients who met the criteria for both fibromyalgia and chronic fatigue syndrome received this vaccine. Improvement among those who received the vaccine was statistically significant, and one year after the study, almost half of the patients who had been unable to work at all prior to the start of treatment were able to return to full or part-time employment. Another study out of Sweden looked at use of staphylococcus toxoid CFS and fibromyalgia, testing 100 different patients. Thirty-three percent of patients had as much as a 50 percent improvement, and treatments over six months led to significant improvement in the patients.

Lymph Node Cell-Based Immunotherapy

A group of top CFS researchers, including Drs. Nancy Klimas, Mary Ann Fletcher, and Roberto Patarca-Montero at the University of Miami, did a study, obtaining lymph nodes from patients and culturing the cells for ten to twelve days with anti-CD3 and interleukin-2m, and then infusing the cells back into the patients, who were followed up for approximately six months. This type of treatment has been shown to facilitate a Th2- to Th1-type cytokine expression shift in some patients. Of the 11 patients in the trial who had cells reinfused, 9 had significant cognitive improvement; other measures of severity of illness also trended toward improvement, with no adverse effects.

Gamma Globulin

Gamma globulin is human immune globulin and contains antibody molecules directed against a broad range of infectious agents. Gamma globulin is typically used as a way to immunize someone with a compromised immune system, or who has been exposed to an infectious agent that has the potential to cause serious disease. Gamma globulin is not considered particularly effective in the treatment of CFS and fibromyalgia, but some practitioners may recommend this treatment.

Isoprinosine/Imunovir

Imunovir is a prescription supplement available outside the U.S. considered to have both immunomodulating and antiviral properties, and registered for the treatment of viral infections. Some research has shown that in particular viral infections, Imunovir—also known as Isoprinosine—can reduce both symptom intensity and duration.

In one study, the use of Imunovir had a significant impact on various cytokine levels and natural killer cell activity, resulting in improvement in symptoms.

In addition to extensive study and use in chemotherapy patients, as a way to prevent viral infection, studies have shown that Immunovir has some ability to slow the progress of AIDS in HIV-infected persons by increasing the number and activity of T cells, T helper cells, and natural killer cells.

While the drug is legal in most countries outside the U.S., special circumstances are needed for use within the U.S. A doctor can contact the manufacturer regarding how to obtain the drug for patients under an FDA "personal use" waiver. The manufacturer, Newport Pharmaceuticals Limited, can be reached in Dublin, Ireland, by telephone at (+353=1=) 890-3011, fax at (+353=1=) 890-3016, Web at *http://www.Newport-pharma.com,* and e-mail at *info@newport-pharma.com*

Ampligen

Ampligen is a synthetic nucleic acid product that was designed to stimulate the production of interferons, a family of immune response modifiers that are also known to have antiviral activity. Ampligen is an immune-modulating drug that is claimed to inhibit viruses and adjust the levels of several key enzymes, both of which ultimately affect the levels of cytokines and lymphokines, chemicals that the immune system uses to communicate with white blood cells regarding immunity. Early research findings shared at the 2001 American Association for Chronic Fatigue Syndrome Conference outlined benefits, including improved cognitive skills, greater vitality, and higher levels of activity. Among severely debilitated CFS patients studied, after twenty-four weeks more than 80 percent of the study participants had significant enough improvements that they entered phase two of the study.

Dr. Richard Podell, who has worked on trials with patients taking Ampligen, told CBS in 2003: "It seems to correct certain subtle metabolic abnormalities that are seen with people who have CFS."

Ampligen is also thought to be able to activate a process by which the enzyme RNase L destroys viral RNA. This is particularly helpful because some of the viruses implicated in CFS and fibromyalgia, such as herpesvirus, reproduce and spread so effectively within the body because they are able to deactivate RNase L.

Some patients treated with Ampligen recovered from serious viral illness. It's not clear, however, whether the drug has the potential to permanently eliminate the conditions, since patients who stopped the drug showed reactivated viruses and again became symptomatic.

Currently, clinical trials are ongoing re: Ampligen, which is only available through those trials. The Food and Drug Administration (FDA) has not yet approved Ampligen for widespread use, and its use is still considered experimental. The drug is fairly difficult to obtain, and very expensive. Approval is expected after trials are completed.

Sizofiran

Sizofiran is an immune-stimulating drug that is derived from the suehirotake mushroom. It's currently being developed as a potential cancer and hepatitis B treatment and studied as a possible CFS treatment.

■ Natural Immune Enhancement

Medicinal Mushroom Supplements

Supplements derived from medicinal mushrooms—in particular, the mycelia mushroom (which includes maitake mushrooms)—have been shown to have immune-enhancing properties. Quality supplements based on these mushrooms have been shown to increase levels of interleukin-12 (IL-12), a powerful cytokine, as well as helping to increase the number and effectiveness of natural killer cells. Among the products most often recommended are Grifron Fraction Maitake, and MGN3.

Juzen-taiho-to

The Japanese herbal medicine Juzen-taiho-to, which is part of a group of Kampo remedies called Hozai, has been shown to help balance Th1/Th2-type responses.

Thymic Protein/Thymic Glandulars

One study found a significant increase in total white blood cell levels among CFS patients taking thymic protein three times a day, along with increases in T suppressor cells, levels of which are usually decreased with CFS.

Thymic glandulars, by providing extracts of healthy tissue from the thymus, lymph, and spleen, appear to help the immune system respond effectively to infection, and are recommended by some alternative practitioners.

Coenzyme Q10

CoQ10 can stimulate the immune system both to kill bacteria, viruses, and parasites, and to increase antibody response.

Vitamin A

Vitamin A helps the immune system by strengthening the mucosal surfaces.

Beta-carotene

Some studies have shown that beta-carotene can help improve natural killer cell activity in some groups. In addition to taking supplements, one may eat red-, orange-, and yellow-colored vegetables, which contain high levels of various carotenes.

Vitamin E

Vitamin E can help immune function and boost natural killer cell activity.

Vitamin C (Ascorbic Acid)

High levels of vitamin C have antioxidant properties and can help boost the immune system.

Vitamin B$_6$ (Pyridoxine)

Vitamin B$_6$ aids immune function.

Quercetin

Quercetin is a powerful flavonoid and antioxidant that has both an anti-inflammatory and an antihistamine effect.

Zinc

Zinc has a role in helping to activate various immune cells, and zinc deficiency can reduce resistance to infection and reduce natural killer cell activity. Zinc also has antiviral properties and significantly reduces the duration of the cold virus.

Copper

A deficiency in copper can impair the lymphocytes' ability to respond to antigens, thereby making the immune system less effective. It's important, however, to ensure that copper is not taken in excess.

According to Ann Louise Gittleman, author of the best-selling book *The Fat Flush Plan*, as well as many leading-edge health books, excess copper—which displaces zinc and can cause zinc deficiency—can be a factor in chronic fatigue syndrome and other immune dysfunctions. Gittleman, a nutritionist, estimates that about three-quarters of her female clients have copper overload, and copper overload, with its corresponding deficiency in zinc, can compromise the immune system:

Copper overload actually is the cause behind the cause of many common health problems, including physical fatigue, mental racing, emotional highs and lows, anxiety, and reproductive problems. Most practitioners don't know anything about it, which is unfortunate because this condition is quite common, especially among women.

Gittleman says women are more prone to copper accumulation because the female hormone estrogen increases copper retention.

Selenium

Selenium is considered immunoprotective as well as antioxidant. Working with Vitamin E, selenium is a potent supporter of proper cell-mediated immunity.

Probiotics

As described in chapter 6, probiotics are the "friendly" or "good" bacteria that help the immune system fight infection, particularly in the intestines. Probiotics help create the optimal environment for enhanced immunity, balance in flora, and the ability to heal in the intestinal linings. A top-quality brand of probiotics, one that at minimum includes billions of live *Lactobacillus acidophilus* and *Bifidobacterium longum* bacteria, is recommended.

Echinacea

Echinacea, which is extracted from the purple coneflower, is considered a natural antiviral and antibiotic, with the ability to fight various viruses and infections, especially the common cold. Echinacea can increase antibody production, reduce inflammation, and enhance the body's cellular ability to fight off infection.

Panax Ginseng

Panax ginseng is an adaptogenic herb that helps the body respond appropriately to stress. Research has shown the ability to enhance natural killer cell function and stimulate cellular immunity. It's considered effective at up-regulating the Th1-type response. Ginseng can have some adverse interactions with prescription drugs, such as warfarin and phenelzine sulfate, among others, so it should only be taken after a professional review of prescribed medications. Experts typically recommend that ginseng not be taken with estrogens or steroid drugs because of possible adverse interactions. Ginseng can have a hypoglycemic effect, and some experts recommend that diabetics not use panax ginseng at all, while others say that close monitoring of blood glucose levels in diabetics is needed.

Grape Seed Extract

Grape seed extract contains chemicals known as proanthocyanidins, which have been found to not only act as a potent antioxidant, but stimulate the immune system and promote the effectiveness of natural killer cells.

L-carnitine

L-carnitine is an amino acid that has shown some ability to help increase natural killer cell activity.

DHEA

Dehydroepiandrosterone (DHEA) is a steroid hormone produced by the adrenal glands that helps to balance and boost the immune system, and promotes healthy balance of other steroid sex hormones such as estrogen and testosterone. DHEA tends to promote a Th1-type response pattern, and may help enhance production of Th1-type cytokines. In one study, DHEA restored normal cytokine production in immune system dysfunction induced by aging. As a hormone, DHEA must be used carefully, under the direction of an expert practitioner, who can monitor serum or salivary levels.

Melatonin

One of the effects of chronic stress and infection is elevated cortisol levels due to overstimulation of the adrenal glands. This excess cortisol is particularly difficult on the immune system. Melatonin, along with DHEA, is effective at helping to suppress cortisol levels. Melatonin is also thought to enhance the production of T-helper cells, which helps fight viruses, bacteria, and other infections. As a hormone, it's particularly important that melatonin use be overseen by a knowledgeable practitioner.

Lifestyle Changes

A variety of lifestyle changes should be incorporated into your plan to enhance your immune system and are described at length in chapter 14. They include, among others,

- Making dietary changes, including reducing or eliminating sugar and high-glycemic simple carbohydrates
- Incorporating good fats—such as those found in olives, avocados, fish, nuts, and seeds—into your diet
- Eliminating or substantially reducing alcohol
- Stopping smoking
- Getting gentle exercise when you can
- Reducing stress
- Avoiding unnecessary vaccinations

8

Endocrine System, Hormones, and the Hypothalamic-Pituitary-Adrenal Axis

> Seeing, hearing, feeling, are miracles,
> and each part and tag of me is a miracle.
> —WALT WHITMAN

Various studies have shown that the body's endocrine system, which produces the body's hormones, and in particular, the hypothalamic-pituitary-adrenal axis (HPA axis) and the thyroid, play a key role in the development of CFS and fibromyalgia.

■ The Hypothalamic-Pituitary-Adrenal (HPA) Axis

The hypothalamic-pituitary-adrenal (HPA) axis is actually just what it sounds like—an endocrine circuit that involves the region of the brain called the hypothalamus, the pituitary gland, and the adrenal glands. As part of the HPA axis, each of these endocrine glands interacts with the others.

The ultimate purpose of the HPA axis is to manage the body's production and release of cortisol.

Cortisol levels fluctuate normally throughout the day, with the highest levels typically seen in the early morning and the lowest levels at midnight. But physical stressors such as sickness, trauma, and surgery or psychological/mental stressors can also trigger a cortisol release. As soon as the body perceives a stressor, the hypothalamus secretes corticotropin-releasing hormone (CRH), which stimulates the pituitary gland. When the pituitary senses CRH, the response is to release adrenocorticotropin-releasing hormone (ACTH). ACTH is also sometimes called corticotropin. The ACTH then goes to the adrenals, via the bloodstream, where it triggers the adrenal gland to release cortisol.

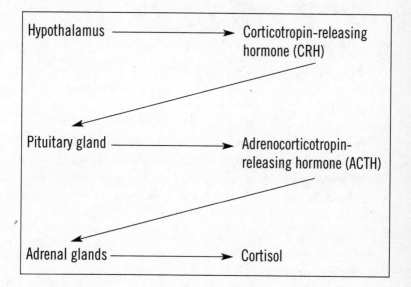

Once cortisol is released, it causes muscle protein to break down, which then releases amino acids into the bloodstream. The liver uses these amino acids to synthesize glucose for energy, raising the blood sugar and diverting energy away from most tissues and toward the brain, in preparation to deal with the stressors.

Cortisol itself also inhibits production of CRH, as part of a negative-feedback loop.

Pituitary and Pineal Glands

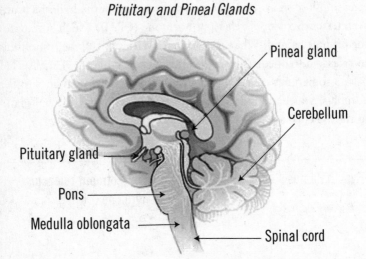

The hypothalamus is the brain's center for controlling appetite, sexual behavior, sleeping, body temperature, and hormones.

The pituitary gland, located just above the roof of the mouth and behind the nose, controls the release of a number of hormones including

- Growth hormone
- Thyroid-stimulating hormone
- Adrenocorticotropic hormone
- Prolactin
- Luteinizing hormone
- Follicle-stimulating hormone
- Antidiuretic hormone
- Oxytocin

The adrenal glands are two small triangular-shaped endocrine glands located on top of each kidney. Each adrenal gland is approximately three inches wide and a half inch high.

Adrenal Gland

Adrenal gland

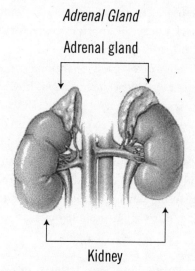

Kidney

Each gland is divided into an outer cortex and an inner medulla. The cortex and medulla of the adrenal gland secrete different hormones. The adrenal cortex is essential to life, but the medulla may be removed with no life-threatening effects. The adrenal cortex consists of mineralocorticoids that are secreted by the outermost region of the adrenal cortex. The principal mineralocorticoid is aldosterone, which acts to conserve sodium ions and water in the body. Glucocorticoids are secreted by the middle region of the adrenal cortex. The principal glucocorticoid is cortisol, which increases blood glucose levels. The third group of steroids secreted by the adrenal cortex is the gonadocorticoids, or sex hormones, including androgens and estrogens.

To meet stressors, the adrenal system not only releases cortisol, but fast-acting adrenaline, which increases heart rate and blood pressure, preparing the body for the familiar "fight or flight" response.

Adrenaline production stops quickly, and under normal circumstances, cortisol levels fall approximately forty-five minutes after the perceived threat is removed.

Physical or emotional stress or trauma are frequently reported prior to the onset of CFS or fibromyalgia. In CFS and fibromyalgia, it's thought by some researchers that the HPA stress response is permanently turned on, leading to chronic excess of cortisol.

Over time, the chronic stimulation of the HPA axis causes the adrenal glands to "burn out," leading to exhaustion, fatigue, poor immunity, and ultimately, reduced levels of cortisol. Since cortisol suppresses inflammation and cellular immune activation, a reduced cortisol level tends to aggravate inflammatory processes.

■ Hormonal, Endocrine, and HPA-Related Conditions

For CFS and fibromyalgia patients, HPA axis disruptions may result in a variety of conditions that can exacerbate existing symptoms and complicate recuperation. Here is a look at some of the more common conditions.

Hypoadrenalism

Hypoadrenalism, or an insufficiency of adrenal hormone production, may contribute in part to the CFS and fibromyalgia processes or symptoms. Research at the National Institute of Mental Health found mild adrenal insufficiency among a majority of CFS patients studied.

Jacob Teitelbaum, M.D., a prominent CFS and fibromyalgia clinician and researcher, in his study of 64 patients with CFS (44 who also had fibromyalgia) showed that 40 had overt or subclinical hypoadrenalism. Says Teitelbaum:

> *One cause may be the hypothalamic master gland not making enough of an adrenal stimulating hormone (CRH). I suspect many people also have adrenal "burnout."*

When the adrenal glands are not functioning optimally, a condition that is known as adrenal fatigue or adrenal exhaustion develops. Some other names for the syndrome include non-Addison's hypoadrenia, subclinical hypoadrenia, hypoadrenalism, and neurasthenia.
Symptoms include

- Excessive fatigue and exhaustion
- Nonrefreshing sleep (you get sufficient hours of sleep but wake fatigued) or sleep disturbances
- Overwhelming inability to cope with stressors
- The feeling of being rundown or overwhelmed
- The craving of salty and sweet foods
- The feeling of being most energetic in the evening
- Low stamina, being slow to recover from exercise
- Slow recovery from injury, illness, or stress
- Difficulty concentrating, brain fog
- Poor digestion
- Low immune function
- Food or environmental allergies
- Premenstrual syndrome or difficulties that develop during menopause
- Consistent low blood pressure
- Extreme sensitivity to cold

Riccardo Baschetti, M.D., has said that CFS and adrenal insufficiency have much in common. Says Dr. Baschetti:

> *[CFS] shares 39 features with primary adrenal insufficiency, including all the physical and neuropsychological symptoms listed in both the original and the revised criteria for Chronic Fatigue Syndrome (CFS), as well as many other abnormalities.*

Conventional practitioners and testing typically cannot diagnose adrenal fatigue because they are prepared only to diagnose extreme dysfunction in the adrenals, such as Addison's disease, a potentially fatal condition in which the adrenals essentially shut down. Holistic or complementary practitioners can do a saliva cortisol test to evaluate adrenal function and diagnose more subtle dysfunctions in the adrenal glands.

Hypothyroidism

Hypothyroidism can result when there is a dysfunction in the overall HPA axis that disrupts the overall balance of the glands, or, more commonly, when there is some sort of immune dysfunction or autoimmune attack on the thyroid gland itself.

Hypothyroidism is considered fairly common in CFS and fibromyalgia patients. Some practitioners, such as Dr. John Lowe, feel that these conditions are actually manifestations of undiagnosed hypothyroidism, or a cellular resistance to thyroid hormone.

In Jacob Teitelbaum's study of 64 CFS patients (44 with fibromyalgia), 30 of the patients had overt or subclinical hypothyroidism.

With an estimated 20,000,000 sufferers—and a vast 13,000,000 of them undiagnosed—hypothyroidism is the most common autoimmune condition in America today, and a very common undiagnosed condition in general. Thyroid disease prevalence increases with age, and generally, women are seven times more likely than men to develop it. A woman faces as high as a one-in-five chance of developing a thyroid problem during her lifetime. The risk of thyroid disease increases with age, and by the age of seventy-four, the prevalence of subclinical hypothyroidism in men, 16 percent, is nearly as high as the 21 percent rate seen in women.

The thyroid is a small bowtie- or butterfly-shaped gland located in the neck, wrapped around the windpipe, and below the Adam's apple area. Considered the master gland of metabolism, the thyroid produces several hormones, of which two are most critical: tri-iodothyronine (T3) and thyroxine (T4). The thyroid has cells that are the only cells in the body capable of absorbing iodine. The thyroid takes in the iodine, obtained through food, iodized salt, or supplements, and combines that iodine with the amino acid tyrosine. The thyroid then converts the iodine/tyrosine combination into the hormones T3 and T4. The "3" and the "4" refer to the number of iodine molecules in each thyroid hormone molecule.

When the thyroid is in good condition, of all the hormones produced by the thyroid, 80 percent will be T4 and 20 percent T3. T3 is considered the biologically more active hormone—the one that actually functions at the cellular level—and is also considered several times stronger than T4. Once released by the thyroid, the T3 and T4 travel through the bloodstream. The purpose is to help cells convert oxygen and calories into energy and serve as the basic fuel of metabolism. As mentioned, the thyroid produces some T3. But the rest of the T3 needed by the body is actually formed from the mostly inactive T4 by a process sometimes referred to as "T4 to T3 conversion." This conversion of T4 to T3 can take place in some organs other than the thyroid, including the hypothalamus, a part of your brain.

The thyroid is part of a huge feedback process in the endocrine system, and is intricately linked to the HPA axis. The hypothalamus in the brain releases something called thyrotropin-releasing hormone (TRH). The release of TRH tells the pituitary gland to release thyroid-stimulating hormone (TSH). This TSH, circulating in your bloodstream, is what tells the thyroid to make thyroid hormones and release them into your bloodstream.

When there is a dysfunction in the HPA axis, the hypothalamus may not release sufficient TRH, which means that even in the presence of thyroid dysfunction, TSH may not elevate, but hypothyroidism can be present.

Common hypothyroidism symptoms include

- Fatigue, exhaustion
- Depression, moodiness, sadness, difficulty concentrating, difficulty remembering
- Sensitivity to cold, cold hands and feet
- Inappropriate weight gain or difficulty losing weight
- Dry, tangled, or coarse hair and hair loss, especially from the outer part of the eyebrow
- Brittle fingernails
- Muscle and joint pains and aches
- Tendonitis in arms and legs, carpal tunnel syndrome
- Plantar fascitis—pain in the sole of the foot
- Swelling or puffiness in the eyes, face, arms, or legs
- Heart palpitations
- Low sex drive
- Infertility, recurrent miscarriages
- Heavy, longer, more frequent, or more painful menstrual periods
- High cholesterol levels, especially when it's unresponsive to diet and medication
- Worsening allergies, itching, prickly hot skin, rashes, hives (urticaria)
- Chronic infections, including yeast infections, oral fungus, thrush, and sinus infections
- Shortness of breath, difficulty drawing a full breath
- Constipation
- Full or sensitive feeling in the neck
- Raspy, hoarse voice

One self-test you can do to potentially detect some thyroid abnormalities is a thyroid neck check. To take this self-test, hold a mirror so that you can see the area of your neck just below the Adam's apple and right above the collarbone. This is the general location of your thyroid gland. Tip your head back, while keeping this view of your neck and thyroid area in your mirror. Take a drink of water and swallow. As you swallow, look at your neck. Watch carefully for any bulges, enlargement, protrusions, or unusual appearances in this area when you swallow. Repeat this process several times. If you see any bulges, protrusions, lumps, or anything that appears unusual, see your doctor right away. You may have an enlarged thyroid or a thyroid nodule, and your thyroid should be evaluated. Be sure you don't get your Adam's apple confused with your thyroid gland. The Adam's apple is at the front of your neck; the thyroid is further down, and closer to your collarbone. Remember that this test is by no means conclusive and cannot rule out thyroid abnormalities. It's just helpful to identify a particularly enlarged thyroid or masses in the thyroid that warrant evaluation.

Another possible sign of thyroid abnormality is a low basal body temperature, which is the temperature taken upon awakening, in bed, before getting up and before any substantial movement. Typically, basal body temperatures lower than 97.8 to 98.2 degrees Fahrenheit are thought by some to potentially indicate hypothyroidism. This self-testing method was popularized by the late Dr. Broda Barnes. Again, this test is not considered conclusive by many practitioners, and does not either definitively diagnose or rule out thyroid abnormalities.

Blood tests are another key way of identifying thyroid problems. The most commonly performed test is the thyroid-stimulating hormone (TSH) test. While ranges vary from lab to lab, the general "normal" range for TSH tests is now from approximately .3 to 3.0—levels above 3.0 are evidence of hypothyroidism and levels below .3 are indicative of hyperthyroidism, although some labs and physicians may still be basing their interpretation on the older normal range values, which were .5 to 5.5.

- If your doctor runs a test called Total T4, or Total Thyroxine, and you had a low thyroxine reading and a high TSH, she or he might consider that indicative of hypothyroidism.
- If your doctor runs a test called Total T4, or Total Thyroxine, and you had a low thyroxine reading and a low TSH, he or she might look into a pituitary problem.
- If your doctor runs a test called Free T4, or Free Thyroxine, and you had a lower than normal level, she or he might consider that indicative of hypothyroidism.
- If your doctor runs a test called Total T3, and your result is normal or below normal, he or she might consider that indicative of hypothyroidism.
- If your doctor runs a test called Free T3, and your results are below normal, she or he might consider that indicative of hypothyroidism.
- Thyroid antibodies tests can also detect the antibodies that signal the presence of autoimmune thyroid disease, even when TSH is normal.

Diagnosis of thyroid disease can be difficult, especially when you have borderline thyroid conditions or when antibodies are present and causing symptoms but bloodwork has yet to reflect the abnormalities. There are practitioners who believe that you do not need to have an elevated TSH level in order to actually be diagnosed and treated for hypothyroidism. Increasingly, innovative doctors are also viewing high-normal or normal TSH levels as possible evidence of low-level hypothyroidism.

If you don't have insurance, or prefer to start with self-testing, you can do a home TSH (thyroid stimulating hormone) test. A company called BIOSAFE received FDA approval for an accurate, affordable (less than $50) home TSH test. BIOSAFE's test kit requires an almost painless finger prick, using their special finger lancet. All you need is a couple of drops of blood, which you put into their collection device and send to BIOSAFE's labs for analysis. Results are mailed back to you quickly. For information or to order a test, you can call BIOSAFE at 1-800-768-8446, extension 123.

Another option is more conventional blood testing, requiring a blood draw from a laboratory, but not requiring a doctor and prescription for the bloodwork. Various companies, including HealthcheckUSA, for example, offer online and telephone ordering of different tests, including standard TSH tests, T4, T3, T3 Uptake, and T4 Total. The tests are priced very affordably, and the services' doctors sign off on bloodwork requests. You typically receive the results directly, online, or by mail.

Ultimately, what is required is a complete clinical evaluation of your thyroid, involving an examination of the thyroid by a professional, who will feel for enlargement, nodules, and masses. Your reflexes will be checked—sluggish reflexes can be a sign of hypothyroidism, and hyperresponsive reflexes are more common in hyperthyroidism. Other clinical details will be observed and family history will be discussed. The clinical observation, in combination with symptoms, plus the results of blood tests should all be taken together to enable diagnosis.

CFS/fibromyalgia expert Dr. Jacob Teitelbaum feels that doctors may need to rely on clinical symptoms—for example, weight gain, fatigue, muscle pains, slow ankle reflexes—to diagnose hypothyroidism. Says Teitelbaum:

The importance of this concept is further supported by newer data that suggests that most patients who are clinically hypothyroid may have normal thyroid blood tests and, when treated with thyroxine, have significant clinical improvement! Indeed, when following thyroid therapy, thought-provoking work by Fraser, et al., suggests the possibility that "biochemical tests of thyroid function are of little, if any, value clinically" and that following clinical signs and symptoms may be more reliable.

Fibromyalgia researcher and practitioner Dr. John Lowe also believes that conventional tests may not be enough, and a trial of thyroid hormone may ultimately be the factor that diagnoses an underactive thyroid. Says Dr. Lowe:

Our studies suggest that perhaps 40% of fibromyalgia patients have "peripheral" tissue resistance to thyroid hormone—not pituitary or general resistance. Patients who have peripheral tissue resistance to thyroid hormone have normal thyroid test results before treatment with thyroid hormone. So, we don't know that they have peripheral resistance until we've treated them.

For those patients who show evidence of thyroid problems or tissue resistance, Dr. Lowe recommends a program he calls "metabolic rehabilitation." He claims to have high levels of success treating fibromyalgia patients with his protocol. According to Dr. Lowe:

When guided properly, patients whose fibromyalgia syndrome is underlain by hypothyroidism and/or thyroid hormone resistance stand a good chance of markedly improving or recovering.

The essential elements of Dr. Lowe's protocol include repeatedly measuring the patient's fibromyalgia status, graphing it, and adjusting the treatment based on this quantification. The primary treatment is thyroid hormone, with a dosage based on changes in objective fibromyalgia measures, the patient's subjective estimate of status, results of a physical examination, and changes in the patient observed by the clinician. The form of thyroid hormone may involve use of levothyroxine, desiccated thyroid (Armour Thyroid), or T3 (Cytomel). The protocol also includes lifestyle practices (such as a healthy diet, nutritional supplements, and exercise to tolerance) that will help aid normalization of the metabolism. As needed, Dr. Lowe also recommends that metabolic rehabilitation include self-care for myofascial trigger points and professional spinal manipulative therapy, and professional mental health support from a practitioner who has experience working successfully with fibromyalgia patients.

One key aspect to Dr. Lowe's protocol that differs from that of many others is his position that patients must eliminate use of narcotic and tranquilizing medications. Says Dr. Lowe:

> *Experience has shown that when the patient is using these and won't or can't give them up, a favorable therapeutic outcome with metabolic rehabilitation is highly unlikely. If the patient intends to continue the use of the medications, there is no point in beginning our protocol.*

Growth Hormone Deficiency

Another endocrine dysfunction that may be related is growth hormone deficiency. Growth hormone is typically replenished during deep sleep, but since deep, restorative stage 4 sleep is often disturbed in CFS and fibromyalgia, this can lead to a growth hormone deficiency.

Symptoms of growth hormone deficiency include fatigue, reduced energy, brain fog and cognitive problems, weak muscles, low exercise tolerance, intolerance to cold, and depression.

One Spanish researcher, Dr. Alfonso Leal-Cerro, reported on his findings at a meeting of the Endocrine Society. Dr. Leal-Cerro said that he has found a high number of fibromyalgia patients who have low levels of insulinlike growth factor 1 (IGF-1). Growth hormone helps increase IGF-1 levels.

FMS expert Robert Bennett, M.D., found that at least one third of his FMS patients meet the criteria for growth hormone deficiency. Another study by Bennett looked at 20 women with fibromyalgia and 10 normal women, putting them through physical stress on a treadmill test. Growth hormone levels went up in the healthy women, but not in the women with fibromyalgia. After giving the women a drug, Mestinon, which blocks somatostatin, a hormone that blocks growth hormone—Bennett had the women take the treadmill test again, and growth hormone levels rose normally, as in the healthy women. Mestinon is used as a myasthenia gravis treatment, but is being looked at for more widespread fibromyalgia treatment.

In another study by Dr. Bennett, 70 female fibromyalgia patients were compared to 55 healthy controls, it was found that stage 4 sleep disruption in the fibromyalgia patients reduced the secretion of growth hormone in the majority of them.

■ Treatments

Low-Dose Hydrocortisone

One treatment advocated by some practitioners for CFS and fibromyalgia patients is low-dose hydrocortisone. Some studies have shown it to have no benefit, but in other cases, particularly where there is evidence of adrenal fatigue, a physiologic replacement dose of hydrocortisone is recommended. One study conducted by British researchers found that giving low doses of hydrocortisone to CFS patients—no more than 5 mg a day—could help relieve fatigue and symptoms without any apparent negative side effects. Experts caution, however, that hydrocortisone therapy is not for everyone, especially people who have high blood pressure, diabetes, cataracts, and certain other conditions.

Hypoadrenalism Recommendations

In addition to low-dose hydrocortisone, there are a variety of other recommendations for hypoadrenalism:

Avoid stimulants. As much as you may want them, stimulants are the equivalent of giving too much gas and "flooding the engine" in a car. It puts further stress on the adrenals to work harder and produce more energy, and ends up further depleting the adrenal glands. Things to avoid include caffeine, guarana, kola nut, and prescription stimulants. Of particular concern is the herbal stimulant ephedra, which can have dangerous side effects for some people.

Balance your blood sugar with your diet. To minimize stress on the adrenal system and ensure maximum energy, consider a low-glycemic (low-sugar) diet consisting of sufficient protein and fat and low-glycemic carbohydrates, eaten in smaller, more frequent meals throughout the day. Sugar and simple carbohydrates put stress on the adrenal glands by rapidly shifting blood sugar levels. By switching to vegetables, fruits, proteins, and high-fiber carbohydrates, you ensure that your blood sugar remains more stable and put less strain on the adrenal glands.

Use adaptogenic herbs for energy. In the book *Living Well with Hypothyroidism*, herbal and aromatherapy expert Mindy Green of the Herbal Research Foundation offers some interesting recommendations about the use of herbs for energy, stimulation, and adrenal support:

> We live in a society that runs on stimulation—whether it's coffee, or violence on television—things that make us live on that edge. So while there are some excellent herbs and essential oils for adrenal support, people need to take care not to try these products along with other stimulants. When you're

trying to tone your adrenals, you don't want to drink caf-
feine, or watch horror movies or violent news stories, for
example. Instead of the simulating effect of aerobics, do
something more calming, like yoga or tai chi. It's almost as if
you need to train your body to run more on internal energy
than outside energy and stimulation.

The way Green describes it is that taking excessive stimulants when
your endocrine or adrenal systems are depleted is "like kicking a
dead horse."

From an herbal standpoint, Mindy recommends Siberian ginseng, as opposed to regular ginseng, and astragalus, which is also
good for immune support, as key tonics for the adrenal and
endocrine systems.

In their book *Herbal Defense*, herbalists Robyn Landis and K. P.
Khalsa discuss the benefits of Siberian ginseng and astragalus, and
also recommend several other herbs for thyroid support:

- Fo-ti root (Ho Shou Wu), a Chinese herb that's broader and
  slower in action than—but similar to—ginseng
- The Ayurvedic remedy Triphala, a long-term glandular tonic
- Black cohosh root, a long-term glandular tonic
- Herbal teas—*not* Coffee

Yerba maté tea. What about coffee fans who are ready to reach
for a double espresso? Try yerba maté tea, pronounced "MAH-tay."
Maté is an herbal tea native to South America. Considered far more
nutritious than black tea or coffee, and though it also has some caffeine, maté typically energizes rather than makes people jittery.

Basic multivitamin/B complex. You will want to take a strong,
balanced formula that provides decent amounts of key factors for
adrenal and metabolic health.

Adrenal glandulars. Desiccated adrenal gland can be helpful to some people in supporting the gland and replacing some missing adrenal hormones. Be sure to get a reputable brand from a reputable supplier to ensure quality, potency, and safety.

Pregnenolone, DHEA. Pregnenolone and DHEA are hormones that can help resolve adrenal fatigue. Use of over-the-counter hormones is recommended only under the guidance of your practitioner.

This is by no means a comprehensive list of supplements or solutions. Your best option is to work with a practitioner to diagnose your adrenal fatigue and to develop a customized treatment program that will help resolve this condition.

Hypothyroidism Treatments

Doctors typically prescribe the synthetic T4 hormone known as levothyroxine to treat hypothyroidism. Popular brands include Levoxyl, Unithroid, Levothroid, and Synthroid. Research reported in the *New England Journal of Medicine* in February 1999, however, found that a majority of patients may feel better on a combination of hormones. On the basis of that study, more doctors are adding synthetic T3 (liothyronine)—the popular brand of which in the U.S. is Cytomel. Other options include time-released, compounded T3, or the drug Thyrolar, which is a synthetic T4/T3 combination. Alternative physicians tend to prefer the natural desiccated thyroid drugs—Armour, Nature-throid, and Biotech—which also include T4 and T3.

Says Dr. John Lowe, fibromyalgia researcher:

My research group has spent the past ten years studying fibromyalgia caused by thyroid hormone resistance. We have laboratory proof that about one third of the fibromyalgia patients we've evaluated and treated have thyroid hormone resistance. Our treatment results have forced us to a firm con-clusion: For most fibromyalgia patients with thyroid hor-mone resistance, using plain T3 (as part of comprehensive metabolic rehab) is the only route to recovery. With the proper use of plain T3, 75% to 85% of these patients perma-nently recover.

Growth Hormone Deficiency

There are two ways to treat growth hormone deficiency. One way is through injections of synthetic growth hormone, and the second method is through the use of HGH secretagogues. These are certain amino acids and other natural HGH releasers that promote or stimulate secretion of HGH.

One study showed that patients who received injections to raise IGF-1 levels began to show improvements at around six months, and even more at nine months.

In a small study in Spain, Dr. Alfonso Leal-Cerro followed 20 women who had both fibromyalgia and low IGF-1 levels. Over a six-month period, women received injections of growth hormone or placebo. The women who received growth hormone had signifi-cantly less morning stiffness and pain and fewer tender points than at the beginning of treatment.

Integrated Treatment

Dr. Jacob Teitelbaum believes that resolving HPA-related condi-tions requires a comprehensive, integrated treatment, including

- Thyroid treatment
- Adrenal support
- Pain and sleep relief
- Antibiotics for bacterial infections
- Treatment for parasites
- Treatment for candida/yeast overgrowth

- Antidepressants for depression, anxiety
- Micronutrient supplementation

Dr. Teitelbaum's research shows that 57 percent of patients had complete resolution of fatigue, and 38 percent had significant but incomplete improvement. Improvements were seen at a median time of seven weeks.

The Brain, Pain, the Nervous System, and the Heart

> For peace of mind, we need to resign
> as general manager of the universe.
> —LARRY EISENBERG

Another area of interest in the search for the reasons behind and triggers for pain and other symptoms in CFS and fibromyalgia is the nervous system—in particular, the brain—as well as heart function. Various researchers theorize that CFS and fibromyalgia are nervous system dysfunctions—manifestations of a condition known as neurally mediated hypotension or "dysautonomia." Some experts believe that the conditions are the result of a difficult-to-diagnose heart condition. It's important to have an understanding of some of these theories.

■ Central Nervous System Dysfunction

One line of thinking points to CFS and fibromyalgia as evidence of a significant disruption in the regulatory mechanisms of the nervous system, or a possible injury to or dysfunction in the brain. It's been demonstrated that most people with fibromyalgia, and many CFS patients, feel intense pain at much lower levels of stimulation than others, and appear to recover from that pain more slowly as well.

In a presentation to the MYOPAIN 2001 conference, one expert, Dr. Manuel Martinez-Lavin, referred to the pain as "sympathetically-maintained pain." This type of pain produces burning, tingling sensations and an overall sensitivity.

Normally, touch or an only mildly painful stimulus, will transmit information to the brain regarding the extent of the touch, or the severity of the pain, and an appropriate response will be sent back by the brain. For example, a light touch would be ignored, whereas if you were touching a hot stove, you'd pull your hand back quickly.

But in fibromyalgia and CFS, even slight stimulation of the nerves can sometimes trigger an inappropriate response that is consistent with the highest degree of pain.

The Pain Process

Feeling pain involves two separate processes in the body. First is the chemical message that is sent to the brain, which interprets the message as the sensation of pain. The second process is the brain's response to that message, releasing chemicals that try to minimize or relieve the pain.

Some experts believe that an imbalance in these chemicals is a critical part of the experience of pain for CFS and fibromyalgia patients.

- Pain stimuli (i.e., physical pressure, inflammation, touching something hot) affect tissue in the body.
- Sensation transfers from the nervous system to the dorsal horn, an area of the spinal cord.
- Spinal cord releases several chemicals, including substance P, a neurotransmitter.

- Chemicals, including substance P, move back out into the body, attempting to bind themselves to neuroreceptors.
- After binding to receptors, chemical messages communicating pain are sent back through the spinal cord to the brain.
- Brain releases neurochemicals—including serotonin, norepinephrine, and natural opiate pain relievers such as enkephalins and endorphins—to the area of the spinal cord where substance P had been released, trying to suppress substance P and minimize the perception of pain.
- When substance P continues to be released, this time alongside suppressive chemicals produced by the brain, two things can happen:
  - Either substance P binds to a receptor and again carries the message of pain back to the brain
  - Or substance P is broken down into two parts—the first part which binds to receptors and produces the sensation of pain, or the other part, which can bind to opposite receptors and inhibit the pain signal and inhibit intact substance P itself

In fibromyalgia or CFS

- Blood levels of substance P may be increased.
- There may be an excess of NMDA (N-methyl-D-aspartic acid), a neurochemical involved in the pain response pathway. Pain produced by NMDA receptors is only slightly blocked by opioids.
- Inhibitor neurochemicals such as serotonin may be deficient. Serotonin is the chemical associated with sleep, mood, movement, appetite, and anxiety. When serotonin is deficient or blocked, this can cause depression, anxiety, irritability, or aggression, among other symptoms.
- GABA may be blocked. GABA (gamma-aminobutyric acid) is a calming and inhibitory brain neurotransmitter that helps prevent

nerve cells from overfiring and can help the body deal with stress and pain messages. Blocking GABA can cause increased pain.

Dr. Daniel Clauw, a professor of medicine at the University of Michigan Medical Center in Ann Arbor, studied functional magnetic resonance imaging (fMRI) brain scans of 16 people diagnosed with fibromyalgia, and 16 controls. During the scans, an instrument periodically applied various levels of pressure to the left thumbnail. The results showed that at the same levels of pressure, fibromyalgia patients had increased blood flow—associated with nerve activity and pain—compared to the control patients. And at different levels of pressure, the fibromyalgia patients reported sensations of pain at half the level of pressure that caused pain among the control group, meaning that fibromyalgia patients apparently have a lower pain threshold.

Dr. Clauw believes these findings demonstrate some sort of central nervous system dysfunction in processing pain signals in people with fibromyalgia.

Ultimately, disordered sleep leads to reduced serotonin, which leads to fewer painkilling endorphins, and a disturbed sympathetic nervous system results in increased pain sensitivity, contributing to CFS and fibromyalgia symptoms.

■ Autonomic Nervous System Dysfunction

Another theory is that CFS and fibromyalgia are the result of autonomic nervous system dysfunctions known as dysautonomias.

Dysautonomia is an imbalance in the autonomic nervous system, the system that controls "unconscious" functions such as heart rate, digestion, and breathing. Within the autonomic nervous system, there's the sympathetic system, which controls the body's "fight or flight" reactions, and the parasympathetic nervous system, which controls the quieter body functions—for instance, the digestive system. Usually, the sympathetic and parasympathetic systems are in balance, but in dysautonomia, they become unbalanced.

In dysautonomia, the sympathetic nervous system produces both epinephrine (also known as adrenaline) and norepinephrine. When nerves activate the inner portion of the adrenal glands, large quantities of epinephrine and norepinephrine can be quickly released into the bloodstream, producing the classic "fight or flight" response, with rapid breathing, rapid blood sugar release, increased muscle tension, improved mental alertness, and slower digestion.

Patient advocate and cardiologist Dr. Richard Fogoros has found that many CFS and fibromyalgia patients complain of dysautonomia symptoms. Says Dr. Fogoros:

> In dysautonomia, the autonomic nervous system loses its balance, and at various times the parasympathetic or sympathetic systems become inappropriately predominant. Symptoms can include frequent, vague but disturbing aches and pains, faintness (or even actual fainting spells), fatigue and inertia, severe anxiety attacks, rapid heartbeat (tachycardia), hypotension (low blood pressure), poor exercise tolerance, gastrointestinal symptoms such as irritable bowel syndrome, sweating, dizziness, blurred vision, numbness and tingling, anxiety and (quite understandably) depression.

Other common dysautonomia symptoms include enhanced pain sensitivity, disturbed sleep, and brain fog.

According to Dr. Fogoros, all of these syndromes are real, honest-to-goodness physiologic (as opposed to psychological) disorders—and probably variants of the same general disorder of the autonomic nervous system.

Some of the autonomic dysfunctions seen include:

• Postural orthostatic tachycardia syndrome (POTS)—where exaggerated heart rate increases by more than 30 beats per minute or above 120 beats per minute within ten minutes of getting out of bed or out of a chair, or what's known in tilt-table testing as a heads-up tilt.

• Neurally mediated hypotension (NMH)—where a drop in blood pressure and an increase in heart rate occur in response to getting out of bed or out of a chair, causing symptoms. This apparently occurs as the body tries to compensate for pooling of blood toward the lower part of the body. One study looking at the connection between NMH and CFS found an abnormal response to a heads-up tilt in 22 of 23 patients with CFS versus only 4 of 14 healthy controls. Another study found that 96 percent of clinically diagnosed CFS patients developed hypotension during a heads-up tilt versus 29 percent of healthy controls.

In both conditions, symptoms include light-headedness, dizziness, nausea, palpitations, tremors, headache, profuse sweating, and fatigue.

■ Heart Problems

Cardiac Viral Infection

Infectious disease specialist Dr. Martin Lerner believes that CFS may be due to an ongoing or reactivated viral heart infection, specifically, Epstein-Barr virus or cytomegalovirus. In two small studies, Dr. Lerner found that 95 percent of CFS patients who were evaluated by Holter monitor testing had subnormal electrocardiograms that showed mild heart damage, compared to 25 percent of healthy subjects.

Lerner himself became ill with CFS in the late 1980s after suffering from viral myocarditis, and since that time he has studied the connection between CFS and viral heart damage, as well as response to antiviral treatment.

According to Lerner, a substantial percentage of patients with CFS who tested positive for Epstein-Barr virus but not cytomegalovirus, and who had had CFS for less than two years, had tremendous improvement in symptoms on a treatment of the antiviral drug valacyclovir for six months. The patients who had both Epstein-Barr virus and cytomegalovirus who received valacyclovir did not improve, however.

Abnormal Heart Pumping

Researcher Arnold Peckerman, M.D., at the VA Medical Center in East Orange, N.J., suspects that a potential heart dysfunction triggering CFS is a blood circulation problem called left ventricular dysfunction. In this condition the main pumping chamber of the heart is weakened, and during and after exercise the heart pumps less blood instead of more, which is typical. Dr. Peckerman tested 16 CFS patients, studying their hearts before and after exercise, and compared the results for four nonathletic controls without CFS. At rest, both the CFS patients and controls showed normal heart pumping. After exercise, however, 13 of the 16 CFS patients' hearts pumped less blood than at rest, compared to increased pumping among the controls. Dr. Peckerman and other researchers suggest that a viral infection may target the heart, causing long-term organ damage and triggering this left ventricular dysfunction. Additional testing is expected to focus on this theory and treatments in CFS.

■ Treatments

Natural Help

A variety of nondrug treatments may help both with the nervous system–driven pain response, and dysautonomia. These approaches include

• **Hydration.** Keeping well hydrated is essential, since dehydration can increase the risk of dysautonomia and nervous system imbalance.

• **Increased salt consumption.** Increasing salt consumption can aid in maintaining increasing blood and fluid volume. This should only be done under your practitioner's supervision, however, because of possible impact on blood pressure.

• **Compression garments.** Wearing compression garments such as support hose or surgical stockings and girdles may help reduce the risk of dysautonomia.

• **Physical activity.** Moderate physical activity every day, whenever possible, is important. It can be particularly helpful in calming and balancing the autonomic nervous system, and minimizing the symptoms and incidence of dysautonomia.

• **Relaxation/stress reduction.** Mindfulness training, biofeedback, and other relaxation and stress reduction techniques may aid in balancing the autonomic nervous system.

• **Avoid stimulants.** It's important to avoid overstimulating the nervous system by taking epinephrine-like substances such as caffeine or ephedra.

• **Eliminating MSG and aspartame.** One study found that eliminating both monosodium glutamate (MSG) and the artificial sweetener aspartame from the diet greatly helped some fibromyalgia patients. The rationale is that both MSG and aspartame are excitotoxins that contain glutamate, which activates the NMDA receptors in the nervous system.

Pain Treatments

Because pain relief is such a critical part of the treatments in CFS and fibromyalgia, here is an overview of the various pain medications you may be prescribed.

Nonopioid analgesics/nonsteroidal anti-inflammatory drugs (NSAIDs). Nonopioid analgesics and NSAIDs (nonsteroidal anti-inflammatory drugs) are considered a first line in pain-relieving drugs for CFS and fibromyalgia pain. Some are available as over-the-counter medications. Examples include aspirin, naproxen (Aleve, Anaprox, Naprosen), ibuprofen (Advil, Bayer Select, Motrin, Nuprin), and piroxicam (Feldene). These medications are generally safe when used as directed, but can have some side effects, including kidney damage, gastrointestinal bleeding and ulcers, abdominal pain, nausea, and vomiting. A newer class of NSAID has been developed, called the Cox-II inhibitors, including celecoxib (CELEBREX), and rofecoxib (VIOXX). (These drugs don't have some of the gastrointestinal side effects seen in the traditional NSAIDS; however, there are also known side effects with these drugs, including some allergies and cold symptoms, among others.)

Strong opioids. Some experts say that fewer than 5 percent of patients require this level of pain control, but many patients report needing opioid pain relievers in order to function optimally. Many combinations of opioids have been effective, as has combining opioids with nonopioids such as aspirin or acetaminophen.

A variety of opioid options exist.

Generic Name	Common Brand Name
Morphine	MSContin, MSIR
Codeine	Tylenol 3 or 4
Propoxyphene	Darvocet, Darvon-N
Oxycodone	OxyContin SR, Roxicodone, Roxicet, Percodan/Percocet
Hydrocodone	Norco, Vicodin
Methadone	Dolophine

Other opioid pain relievers include

- Hydromorphone hydrochloride (such as Dilaudid)
- Fentanyl (such as Duragesic)
- Buprenorphine (such as Buprenex)

There are some side effects to opioid medications, including

• **Nausea, vomiting.** Some physicians will prescribe a nonprescription antinausea medication such as Bonine or Dramamine, or a prescription medication such as prochlorperazine (Compazine) or haloperidol (Haldol). Usually this side effect will subside after a few days.

• **Dizziness/sleepiness.** These can be fairly common on opioid therapy, however people on opioids for chronic pain management often develop tolerance and do not have this side effect.

- **Constipation.** This is one of the most common problems for everyone, and typically does not go away. Regular use of laxatives may be necessary in order to ensure regular bowel movements.
- **Respiratory depression.** The most dangerous side effect of opioids is their ability to suppress breathing. Typically, however, this requires either an overdose in someone using the drugs for chronic pain or a high dose in people who are not in pain and are abusing the drugs. For a chronic pain patient, increased dosages of opioids, when prescribed under a physician's supervision, will not cause respiratory depression.
- **Addiction.** A key issue regarding opioids is that relatively higher doses are needed over time in order to relieve pain. This raises the concern for addiction. Many studies, however, have shown that when properly managed, use of opioids is safe and rarely addictive. People in chronic pain can take high doses without the same side effects as people who are not in pain and abuse these drugs. Addiction also seems to primarily afflict those who already show addictive behavior. In one study, 12,000 nonaddicted people who needed opioids were followed up to see if they had become addicted, and only four—less than a tenth of 1 percent—showed evidence of subsequent addiction.

Antidepressants have proven to be particularly helpful with CFS and fibromylagia pain. Antidepressants such as selective serotonin reuptake inhibitors (SSRIs) enable the brain to maintain slightly higher levels of serotonin, and higher serotonin regulates the brain's ability to control pain and modulate mood, motivation, sleep, and behavior. Tricyclic antidepressants such as amitriptyline (Elavil) can help increase levels of natural opiates, endorphins. New antidepressants in the pipeline will include a variety of drugs that will act as "substance P blockers," as well as corticotropin-releasing hormone (CRH) blockers.

Some patients may be reluctant to take an antidepressant for pain, thinking that it is stigmatized in some way or is only for people who have mental health problems. Kathy was one of those patients:

About 2 years ago, I started taking Zoloft. I was very hesitant about taking it, because it is an antidepressant drug. I was upset about taking it because I felt like the nurse practitioner told me that I was NOT depressed, and explained about the benefits of Zoloft helping with my severe and excruciating pains. So I went ahead and started taking the Zoloft. After a couple of weeks, about 90% of my pain was GONE, and the remaining pain was tolerable—mild. Now NO ONE can take the Zoloft away from me. It has greatly relieved my pain. So I continue with 50mg of Zoloft every evening. IT WORKS! I know many people don't like taking antidepressants, but give it a try! The pain is real, and this will really help. The same neural transmitters that control our moods, ALSO controls our pain reception. So don't hesitate like I did. Take it, so you can receive relief sooner.

One promising treatment being reviewed is milnacipran, developed for the treatment of fibromyalgia and other chronic pain disorders. Milnacipran is the first of a new type of drugs called norepinephrine serotonin reuptake inhibitors (NSRIs). This makes it similar to the antidepressant venlafaxine (Effexor) which is a serotonin norepinephrine reuptake inhibitor (SNRI). The fact that milnacipran's reuptake is preferential to norepinephrine means that it may be particularly suited to chronic pain, and may function similarly to tricyclic antidepressants, with fewer side effects. In phase 2 trials, milnacipran was shown to provide statistically significant improvement of pain in fibromyalgia patients. As many as 37 percent of the patients treated twice a day with milnacipran reported at least a 50 percent reduction in pain intensity, compared to 14 percent of patients who received a placebo. The milnacipran-treated patients also had less fatigue and reduced depression.

A variety of other drugs and supplements may be of help in treating pain:

• **Pregabalin.** One interesting and promising treatment under investigation is the drug Pregabalin. Preliminary tests have shown that Pregabalin is safe, and may help improve pain, sleep quality, fatigue, and other symptoms in fibromyalgia patients. Pregabalin is a drug that may help prevent the blocking of GABA, resulting in pain relief, among other symptoms. In a research study of fibromyalgia patients, patients treated with Pregabalin at a level of 450 mg per day experienced as much as a 50 percent reduction in pain over time, compared to the start of the study.

• **Antiseizure medications, like gabapentin (Neurontin) and clonazepam (Klonopin).** These can help with nervous system imbalances and pain.

• **5-HTP supplementation.** The amino acid tryptophan is converted into 5-hydroxytryptophan (5-HTP), which ultimately becomes the neurotransmitter serotonin. Supplementation with 5-HTP may be a help in raising serotonin levels in some people.

• **L-theanine supplementation.** The amino acid L-theanine, a component of green tea, can increase levels of GABA. L-theanine appears to have a role in forming GABA.

• **Beta blockers.** Drugs such as atenolol (Tenormin) and propranolol hydrochloride (Inderal) can reduce adrenaline output from the adrenals, helping to interrupt the pain process.

Dysautonomia

A number of drug therapies may be able to help with dysautonomia, including

- **Drugs for low blood pressure.** The drug fludrocortisone acetate (Florinef) improves low blood volume. Fludrocortisone is a steroid drug used to help maintain the balance of certain minerals and water for good health.

- **Stimulants.** A variety of stimulant drugs also help constrict blood vessels, reverse low blood pressure, and reduce blood pooling, including methylphenidate (Ritalin, Concerta), dextroamphetamine (Dexedrine), midodrine (ProAmatine)

- **Antidepressants.** According to cardiologist Richard Fogoros, M.D., there is some evidence that antidepressants might actually help to "rebalance" the autonomic nervous system in some patients. Selective serotonin reuptake inhibitors (SSRIs) such as fluoxitine (Prozac), sertraline (Zoloft), and paroxetine (Paxil) have been helpful for postural orthostatic tachycardia syndrome and other dysautonomia syndromes. And tricyclic antidepressants such as amitriptyline (Elavil) and nortriptyline (Pamelor) have been shown to be helpful at low doses for some cases of dysautonomia.

- **Cardiac medications.** Heart medications such as beta blockers—for example, atenolol (Tenormin)—calcium blockers, and antiarrhythmic drugs have been helpful with some dysautonomia symptoms.

- **Anti-anxiety/antiseizure drugs.** Medications such as alprazolam (Xanax), lorazepam (Ativan) and clonazepam (Klonopin) may help with some of the anxiety-related symptoms of dysautonomia in some patients.

Sensitivities, Allergens, and Toxins

> **Man is a complex being: he makes**
> **the deserts bloom and lakes die.**
> —GIL STERN

Another direction experts look to in terms of factors that play a key role in CFS and fibromyalgia is the area of chemical sensitivities and overexposure or sensitivity to various toxins and allergens.

■ Sensitivities/Allergies

Chemical Exposure

Some studies have shown that a significant percentage of people with CFS and fibromyalgia show sensitivity to various chemicals and pollutants, including pesticides, cigarette smoke and fumes from gasoline, paint, solvents, nail polish remover, ammonia cleaners, perfumes, hair spray, carpeting, dry cleaning, and other exposures. There are also anecdotal reports of the onset of CFS and fibromyalgia after an incident of overexposure to a toxin. Some of these substances are known to act as poisons in the brain, and it is this mechanism that may be at work in CFS and fibromyalgia. Some toxins can have an impact on NMDA (N-methyl-D-aspartate), and therefore can interrupt the proper functioning of the pain receptor process.

Symptoms of chemical sensitivity include brain fog, mood disorder, and respiratory problems such as asthma, shortness of breath, runny nose, and headaches. The symptoms usually begin fairly quickly, within minutes after the exposure to the triggering chemical or toxin.

One clue that you may be chemically sensitive is that you have a strong dislike—or *like*—of various smells, including gasoline fumes, fresh paint, cigarette smoke, or dry cleaning solvents.

Mercury/Metals

Another theory as to the cause of CFS and fibromyalgia is toxic overexposure to metals. Some practitioners are concerned about mercury poisoning in particular, and some holistic practitioners recommend avoiding mercury-loaded fish and, in some cases, even removal of mercury amalgam tooth fillings.

Dale Guyer, M.D., whose practice focuses in part on CFS and fibromyalgia patients, has said that nine out of ten times his patients with CFS and fibromyalgia have elevated levels of toxic metals, based on challenge tests. Not only does he find mercury, but also lead, cadmium, and arsenic.

Food Allergies/Sensitivities

Food allergies and sensitivities have been implicated as potential contributors to the CFS and fibromyalgia process.

One small study, conducted by Dr. Joel S. Edman of the Center for Integrative Medicine at Thomas Jefferson University Hospital in Philadelphia, Pennsylvania, found that people with fibromyalgia might actually have a reduction in symptoms when they eliminate allergenic foods from their diet. Patients removed common allergens from their diet, and after two weeks without eating any of the allergens, almost half of the patients reported a significant reduction in pain, and more than three-fourths had a reduction in symptoms such as headache, fatigue, bloating, heartburn, and breathing difficulties.

Some of the most common allergenic foods include

- Wheat
- Dairy foods
- Corn
- Soy
- Fish (especially shellfish)
- Nuts
- Fruits

Some practitioners believe that unsuspected and unidentified allergenic reactions may cause inflammation and contribute to the overall immune dysfunction that sets CFS and fibromyalgia in motion.

The mechanism by which this happens may be the so-called "leaky gut syndrome," in which food allergies inflame the intestinal lining, allowing large protein molecules to leak through the intestinal membrane and into the bloodstream. There these proteins are perceived as invaders, and they activate the immune system. In leaky gut syndrome, this process goes on continually.

To find out if you have food allergies, you can have food allergy testing, either conventional skin testing or the more elaborate and sensitive IgG4 and IgG1 (delayed) food allergy testing via blood test.

The least expensive option is to try an elimination diet, where you remove various foods from your diet, and then reintroduce them, noting symptomatic reactions. To do an elimination diet, you need to remove an item completely from your diet for two weeks. Then eat a large amount of the food you're testing to see if you have any noticeable reaction over the next seventy-two hours. You're looking for diarrhea, nausea, gas, headache, rashes, skin eruptions, itching, fatigue, irritability, and other strong reactions or symptoms.

One of the most common food sensitivities linked to autoimmune diseases—and therefore a possible risk factor for CFS and fibromyalgia—is sensitivity to gluten, a protein found in the grains of wheat, rye, and barley. In its full expression it can cause celiac disease—complete intolerance to gluten products. But even sensitivity to gluten may contribute to immune dysfunction. One proponent of this theory is Dr. James Braly, an author, lecturer, and researcher who argues that human beings have strayed far from the diet we originally subsisted on animal proteins, as well as fruits and vegetables. It was only until relatively recently on the human time line that grains were introduced. Yet gluten is now one of our most common foods, and even the newly revised food pyramid advises people to eat six to eleven servings of grains each day. Says Dr. Braly:

> We've gone from being hunter-gatherers to being canaries. Yet our society's dependence on gluten may not at all be healthy. From 20 to 30 percent of the population actually has undiagnosed, untreated gluten sensitivity, which manifests itself in a variety of health problems.

Dr. Braly says the gluten sensitivity and celiac disease linkage needs to be ruled out in the case of a number of diseases, including fibromyalgia. Dr. Braly feels that it's worth evaluating because there's hope you can lessen the symptoms, possibly eliminate the need for medication, and prevent other diseases from occurring.

■ Neurotoxins

A neurotoxin is anything that has a poisonous effect on nerves and nerve cells. By affecting the nervous system negatively, these poisons can have an impact on the pain process and other pathways that contribute to CFS and fibromyalgia development and symptoms. Some experts believe that CFS and fibromyalgia may be part of a larger grouping of "chronic neurotoxin-mediated illnesses," caused by exposure to biotoxins.

Excitotoxins

Certain foods are known to act as excitotoxins, which are molecules that excite neurotransmitters and can lead to nerve toxicity when you are overexposed. Two excitotoxins that are potentially linked to CFS and fibromyalgia are monosodium glutamate (MSG) and the artificial sweetener aspartame (NutraSweet). One study found that eliminating MSG and aspartame from the diet of several fibromyalgia patients resulted in dramatic symptom improvement.

Ciguatoxin/Fish Toxins

A neurotoxin that is getting quite a bit of attention among CFS researchers is ciguatoxin, which is a poison that is acquired by warm-water reef tropical ocean fish and then passed on to people who eat the fish, or who eat chickens or fish that are fed such fish. The poisoned fish have eaten particular types of algae that do not degrade and are toxic in people. Ciguatoxin poisoning—known as ciguatera—is actually the most common nonbacterial, fish-borne poisoning in the United States.

The most common types of fish implicated are grouper, amberjack, red snapper, eel, sea bass, barracuda, and Spanish mackerel. Ciguatoxin is not affected by cooking, and you cannot tell by smelling or looking at the fish whether it is poisoned by ciguatoxin.

The majority of ciguatera outbreaks in the United States occur in Hawaii and Florida, although the increasing export of warm-water fish around the world has meant that ciguatera can occur almost anywhere.

Researchers have found ciguatoxin in the blood of CFS patients. Symptoms of ciguatera include neurological problems such as pain, burning, tingling and numbness in limbs, headache, dysautonomia, gastrointestinal distress, muscle pain, and other symptoms.

At the 2002 International Symposium on Toxins and Natural Products in Okinawa, Japan, Dr. Yoshitsugi Hokama, a worldwide expert on fish toxins, reported on his research into ciguatoxin. Dr. Hokama found that all the CFS patients he tested had evidence of ciguatoxin exposure, and some CFS patients had higher levels than even patients with acute ciguatera.

Another fish toxin that may be implicated in CFS and fibromyalgia is pfiesteria, the "fish-killer" toxin that is found in some rivers and bays.

Blood tests can diagnose some neurotoxin exposure. Other experts use controversial visual contrast sensitivity testing, which is thought to be able to detect the quality-of-vision issues that show up after overexposure to neurotoxins.

■ Treatments

Avoiding Exposure

Avoiding exposure to allergens, toxins, or irritants is one of the first lines of defense:

• For food allergens, identify the foods that trigger allergic symptoms (via testing, or via a rotation diet), and consider removing trigger foods from your diet entirely.

- Avoid eating fish that are known to be particularly high in metals. Dr. Joseph Mercola, author of *The No-Grain Diet,* says that the only "safe" fish from the standpoint of metal toxicity are summer flounder, wild Pacific salmon, croaker, sardines, haddock, and tilapia.

- Rotate your diet. Don't eat the same food every day. Try to give yourself three or four days before repeating foods to avoid overexposure that can trigger allergies.

- Switch to natural pesticides and natural cleaning products, pay extra for full service at the gas station, or make other modifications that allow you to minimize exposures to toxic fumes and chemicals.

- Dust-proof your bedroom by getting rid of wall-to-wall carpets and down-filled comforters and pillows. Get rid of carpeting in the bathroom.

- Regularly wash bedding and curtains, dust furniture, and damp-mop floors to remove dust and kill dust mites.

- Get an airtight, dustproof plastic cover for your mattress.

- Keep animals out of your bedroom.

- Use an HEPA (high-efficiency particulate air) filter in your bedroom and the main rooms of your house. These filters can remove most airborne allergens.

- Use a vacuum fitted with an HEPA filter to avoid spreading allergens around.

- Minimize mold by keeping humidity low with a dehumidifier or air conditioner. Use an exhaust fan or open windows in the bathroom. A squeegee can help remove excess water from wall surfaces in the bathroom. Remove visible mold from walls, ceilings, and tile surfaces in the bedroom and bathroom, and use mold-killing, mold-preventing cleaners.

Detoxification for Chemical Exposure and Metals

Detoxification is a complicated area, and selecting and following the right detoxification program requires that you work with a practitioner who has expertise in managing patient "detox." Also keep in mind that while detoxing you may not have as much energy as usual, so you will likely want to avoid particularly strenuous exercise and make sure you get enough sleep to support your detox process.

Whatever type of detox you are doing, you can also support it by

- Regular soaks in Epsom salts, baking soda, sea salts, or other detoxifying agents
- Skin brushing, to remove toxins from the skin
- Stretching, relaxation, breathing, and stress-reduction exercises
- Massage and manual drainage, to detox the lymphatic system
- Saunas, which have been shown to help remove fat-stored toxins

Here is an overview of some of the most popular detox approaches:

Fasting detox. A fasting detox typically involves drinking only water, or in the case of a "juice fast," vegetable and/or fruit juices. A one-day or several-day fasting detox, including in particular lemon juice and olive oil, can help support the liver in active detoxification. Fasting is sometimes combined with enemas or bowel-cleansing protocols to help clean out the bowels and eliminate bacteria and toxins in the intestinal tract.

Dietary detox. Basic to all dietary detoxing is two key principles:

- Eat organic, hormone-free, pesticide-free foods whenever possible.
- Drink filtered water.

From that point, dietary detox may involve eating one type of food for several days (a particular fruit, or rice, etc.) and can have some benefits in terms of calming down the immune system and aiding the liver in detoxing. Another type of dietary detox is to go to only fresh fruits and vegetables and whole grains, with no animal, dairy, or nuts. Another level of dietary detox is an all fruits and vegetables diet. All raw foods can be a help to some as a detox regimen—featuring sprouted greens and grains, nuts, fruits, and vegetables, with nothing cooked. Other specialized detox diets include macrobiotic regimens, antiyeast/candida diets, and special allergy diets.

Colon therapy. Colonic irrigation—known as a "colonic"—can help clean out toxins from the intestines. Some practitioners and patients are dedicated to this particular detox method and claim that it helps remove toxins from the body and results in improved well-being.

Lymphatic drainage. The lymph system is one of the body's waste filters, and various practitioners have found that massage, osteopathic and chiropractic lymph drainage techniques, as well as vigorous aerobic exercise, can speed up lymphatic flow, which helps to reduce swelling and pull out waste products for elimination and detoxification.

Chelation therapy. In chelation therapy, the synthetic amino acid EDTA (ethylenediaminetetraacetic acid) is given intravenously. EDTA binds to toxic metals and is then flushed out of the body via the kidneys. A variety of supplement-based oral chelating formulas and regimens are also popular with various practitioners. These vary by practitioner, and you would need to work with your practitioner to determine the optimum therapy for you.

Herbal detox. A number of herbs are known to aid in the detoxification process. The right selection and balance of herbs is up to your practitioner to determine, based on your particular health situation. Cleansing herbs include garlic, red clover blossoms, echinacea, dandelion root, chaparral, cayenne pepper, ginger root, licorice root, yellow dock root, burdock root, sarsaparilla root, prickly ash bark, oregon grape root, parsley leaf, and goldenseal root.

Conventional Allergy Treatments

Some of the conventional allergy treatments that may be of help include the following:

- **Immunotherapy/desensitization shots.** These are the "allergy shots" that many people have had as children and teenagers to help reduce sensitivity to particular allergens. There is evidence that these can be help in some cases, but may not be effective for all people or allergens.
- **Antihistamine drugs.** Over-the-counter and prescription antihistamines such as Benadryl, loratadine (Claritin, Alavert), desloratadine (Clarinex), fexofenadine (Allegra), and ceterizine (Zyrtec) may be of help in controlling allergic response, particularly for environmental and seasonal allergies. Benadryl is considered particularly effective in severe allergic responses since it is quite fast acting.
- **Cromolyn sodium (Nasalcrom) spray.** Some practitioners recommend the cromolyn sodium sprays, which when used over time can help reduce reactivity to inhaled allergens with few side effects.
- **Steroid nasal sprays.** Steroid nasal sprays such as Vancenase, Beconase, and Flonase can be particularly effective for severe nasal allergies. However, they do run the risk of some steroid side effects.

Natural Treatments for Allergies

There are a number of natural allergy treatments that can be incorporated into a CFS or fibromyalgia patient's self-care regimen:

- **Probiotics.** Imbalances of intestinal bacteria are frequently seen alongside allergies, and some allergies actually originate with the membranes of the intestinal system—the gut. A good-quality probiotic supplement is an essential part of any program to deal with sensitivities and allergies.

- **Nasal washing/neti/saline sprays.** One way to keep allergens out of the nasal passages is a practice known as nasal washing, or, to yoga practitioners, neti. This involves running warm salt water into the nasal passages in order to rinse away any irritants. There are devices that you can use for nasal washing, the most basic being a "neti pot," sold with yoga supplies. The neti pot looks like a small Aladdin's lamp. You fill the pot with water and salt and pour into the nostrils one at a time. The saline solution goes into one nostril, crosses to the other, and is expelled in one long stream. A similar effect to nasal washing and neti can be obtained by using hydrating saline nasal sprays.

- **Lower-protein diets.** A lower-protein diet, especially one that eliminates cow's milk and milk products, may help in reducing allergenic response, since milk proteins are common allergens, particularly affecting the respiratory tract and mucous membranes.

- **Quercetin.** Quercetin is a bioflavonoid supplement derived from buckwheat and citrus fruit. Quercetin works as an anti-inflammatory, and calms and stabilizes the cells that release histamine. It works as a preventative, so it needs to be taken regularly, over a period of weeks, before exposure to the allergen.

- **Cayenne pepper.** Some practitioners recommend using cayenne pepper on food or as supplements, claiming that its ingredient, capsaicin, is particularly effective as an allergy treatment.

- **High-dose Vitamin C.** High-dose Vitamin C (basically, vitamin C to bowel tolerance) is reported by some practitioners to have a dramatic effect on allergy symptoms due to its anti-inflammatory effects.

Nambudripad Allergy Elimination Technique (NAET)

NAET stands for Nambudripad allergy elimination technique, a controversial but interesting technique that practitioners claim helps diagnose and treat allergies. The technique named for Dr. Devi S. Nambudripad, its originator, combines the muscle response testing of kinesiology with chiropractic and acupressure techniques to clear allergic reactions by reprogramming the brain's response to allergens. Recipients of NAET treatment claim dramatic reduction or elimination of allergy symptoms after a series ten to twenty sessions. NAET is based on the theory that symptoms can result when allergic responses disrupt energy flows and pathways. The aim of NAET is to desensitize the response to allergens. In NAET, small vials filled with various allergens are placed in the patient's hand, and muscle response testing is used to determine sensitivities. Once the various allergens are identified, treatment involves holding a vial of the allergen while particular acupuncture points are stimulated. This technique is supposed to clear the sensitivity, and if the allergen is avoided for twenty-four hours, it is claimed, the sensitivity will be gone.

Neurotoxin Treatment

One treatment for neurotoxin overexposure is the drug cholestyramine (CSM), a cholesterol-lowering drug that has been in use for more than two decades. The drug binds cholesterol—and in an as-yet unknown mechanism also binds to biological toxins—and excretes them safely.

One study found that pfiesteria patients who took CSM improved, compared to patients taking a placebo. Anecdotally, the CSM treatment is also being used successfully in Lyme disease, chronic ciguatera poisoning, brown recluse spider bites, and other toxic conditions.

Nutritional Imbalances and the "Guai" Protocol

We are indeed much more than what we eat,
but what we eat can nevertheless help us to be
much more than what we are.

—ADELLE DAVIS

Some experts believe that nutritional and enzyme deficiencies and imbalances are at the heart of CFS and fibromyalgia.

■ Magnesium

One theory is that magnesium deficiency plays a role in CFS and fibromyalgia. Magnesium is a mineral needed for immune system function and metabolism. Magnesium deficiencies are known to cause various symptoms, including fatigue, pain, sleep disruption problems, mitral valve prolapse, and other symptoms.

In one study of fibromyalgia patients, a researcher found that 80 percent took a multivitamin, and the next most popular supplement among patients was calcium, which was being taken by 76.5 percent of the patients surveyed. When asked which supplement they considered the most effective for fibromyalgia symptoms, the hands-down winner was magnesium, with almost 30 percent of the votes. Calcium was second, with only 18.7 percent of patients reporting that as their favorite. Said study author Dr. Daniel Wagner, ". . . [A]ll of the vitamin/herbal supplements showed only 20% effectiveness or less. The lone exception to the reported effectiveness of both drugs and supplements was magnesium, which was reported to be almost 30% effective. In general, it is my top recommendation for FMS."

■ L-carnitine

L-carnitine is an amino acid that is an essential part of energy production at the cellular, mitochondrial level. In one study of l-carnitine levels in thirty-five patients with CFS, all had significantly lower l-carnitine levels than normal, and the level of deficiency was statistically proportional to the degree of fatigue reported by the patient. Japanese researchers also found that most patients with CFS studied showed a low level of serum acetylcarnitine, and that the levels also correlated with the level of fatigue experienced.

Some research has even shown supplementation with l-carnitine to help—particularly with fatigue—in as many as 50 percent of those people with CFS studied.

■ Choline

Researchers using state-of-the-art brain-scanning technology looked at a group of patients with CFS, compared to a group of healthy controls. They found higher-than-normal levels of choline, which creates an abnormality of metabolism in the brain in the CFS patients, theorizing that this may be a key factor in the condition. Choline controls the levels of fat in brain cells, and creatinine provides energy. The researchers believe that an imbalance in choline causes abnormal phospholipid metabolism. Phospholipids are types of fats that are an essential part of cells, and they are protected by certain fatty acids. The researchers studying choline imbalances also suggested that taking fatty acid/fish oil supplements that are high in eicosapentaenoic acid (EPA) might help to address the imbalance and alleviate some symptoms.

■ B_{12}

A variety of anecdotal reports and some published studies have shown that people with CFS have improvement in symptoms and energy when given vitamin B_{12} injections. B_{12} reportedly can help with numbness, tingling, and weakness in the hands and feet, memory loss, and fatigue associated with B_{12} deficiency. Patients appeared to respond with in twelve to twenty-four hours after receiving injections of 2,000–2,500 mcg, with improved energy and well-being lasting as long as two to three days. CFS expert Dr. Charles Lapp recommends injections of 3,000 mcg of the cyanocobalamin form of B_{12} every two to three days for his patients. He has reported that an informal poll of his patients showed that 50 to 80 percent felt there was some improvement linked to B_{12} injections, despite their having started with normal B_{12} levels prior to the treatment. Most patients on regular B_{12} therapy learn to do the injections themselves, so they can administer the several injections per week needed to follow this particular treatment protocol.

■ Multivitamins

Dr. Jacob Teitelbaum believes that nutritional deficiencies need to be considered and treated, but not in isolation. Instead, he sees the deficiencies as part of an overall picture that includes hormonal deficiencies, opportunistic infections, and sleep disorders. A foundational aspect of Dr. Teitelbaum's treatment approach for both CFS and fibromyalgia is a daily regimen of a comprehensive and lengthy list of recommended nutrients, which are described at length in his book *From Fatigued to Fantastic,* and listed at his Web site. He has created a powder-form vitamin that can be mixed into a drink, and when accompanied by a B-complex capsule, the drink provides fairly complete nutritional supplementation for CFS and fibromyalgia patients, according to Dr. Teitelbaum. The only supplemental nutrients that he feels can be important but are not included in the supplement are calcium and iron, due to their ability to interact with thyroid hormone absorption and because patients likely want control over the amount of calcium to take and whether or not they need iron.

Another approach that some practitioners have found helpful is the "Myers cocktail," an intravenous therapy of vitamins and minerals that is reported to be effective in treating a variety of problems, including migraine headaches, chronic fatigue syndrome, allergies, heart disease, asthma, fibromyalgia, infections, and numerous other conditions. The Myers cocktail, created more than three decades ago by John Myers, M.D., contains magnesium, calcium, vitamin B_{12}, vitamin B_6, vitamin B_5, vitamin B complex, and vitamin C in high concentrations. The Myers cocktail is a prescription treatment that must be given by a trained practitioner.

■ Phosphate Excess: The Guaifenesin Protocol

R. Paul St. Amand, M.D., is author of one of the most popular and controversial books on fibromyalgia, *What Your Doctor May* Not *Tell You About Fibromyalgia: The Revolutionary Treatment That Can Reverse the Disease*. In his book Dr. St. Amand, an assistant clinical professor at the UCLA School of Medicine, outlines his discovery of and recommended protocol for use of the drug guaifenesin as a treatment for fibromyalgia.

Dr. St. Amand's protocol is based on the theory that a genetic defect changes the kidney's ability to handle phosphate. Phosphate is a compound of phosphorus, a major mineral that is needed for proper DNA/RNA structure and for cellular energy. According to St. Amand, the body begins to accumulate phosphate, and to a lesser extent, calcium, until these minerals start to overwhelm the body at a cellular level. The cells and their mitochondria, which create energy, then become dysfunctional and unable to produce sufficient energy, which Dr. St. Amand believes leads to fibromyalgia symptoms.

The protocol is based on the use of guaifenesin, which is an ingredient in many cold and cough medicines that helps liquefy mucus.

The point of the "guai" protocol is actually to worsen the symptoms. According to Dr. St. Amand's approach, when symptoms worsen, or new symptoms appear, this is evidence that reversal of fibromyalgia has started.

In Dr. St. Amand's guaifenesin protocol, the location, size, and degree of hardness of swellings within the muscles, tendons, and ligaments are mapped. This map, in combination with patients' own reports of fatigue and pain symptoms, serves as a baseline for measuring of progress.

Dosage generally begins with 300 mg (one-half tablet) of time-released guaifenesin two times per day for a week. If they feel far worse at this dosage, this is the optimal dosage, which is the case for approximately 20 percent of patients, according to Dr. St. Amand.

At the end of the week, if symptoms have not gotten worse, the dosage is upped to 600 mg twice a day. As many as 50 percent will begin reversing at this dosage level.

An additional 30 percent of patients need to go to higher doses, and they slowly raise their dose over time until they see the worsening of symptoms that is a sign of reversal.

At 1,800 mg daily, as many as 90 percent of people have found their proper cycling dose, according to Dr. St. Amand, and only 10 percent of patients need to go as high as 2,400 mg a day.

As reversal continues, symptoms improve.

Dr. St. Amand's rough formula is that two months of proper guaifenesin treatment can potentially reverse at least one year of accumulated disease.

Avoiding Salicylates

An important part of Dr. St. Amand's protocol focuses on the avoidance of salicylates.

One of the key aspects of the protocol, and the one that can prove difficult for some patients in implementation, is complete avoidance of internal or external use of aspirin and any aspirin compounds, including salicylate or salicylic acid. Salicylates, found in most plant materials, are easily absorbed through the skin and intestines, but since they have the ability to totally block the effects of guaifenesin, they need to be avoided entirely.

This sounds fairly straightforward—however, these compounds are quite common in many products, all of which have to be faithfully avoided, according to Dr. St. Amand, in order to see results from the protocol.

Dr. St. Amand's book, Web site, and support lists provide greater detail on how to avoid salicylates, but a list of some of the products that need to be avoided entirely while on the protocol include

- Pain medicines that contain aspirin, salicylate, or salicylic acid. (Pain medications such as acetaminophen [Tylenol], ibuprofen [Advil, Aleve], or other nonsteroidal anti-inflammatory drugs are not a problem, nor are narcotics such as codeine and hydrocodone [Vicodin], since they do not block guaifenesin.)
- Many pain creams and lotions such as BENGAY, MYOFLEX, capsaicin
- Alka-Seltzer
- Many herbal medications, including ginseng, Saint-John's-wort, ginkgo biloba, saw palmetto, algae, echinacea, or noni juice, alfalfa, anything with rose hips or bioflavonoids
- Wart- and callus-removal products
- Many acne products
- Skin creams and lotions
- Sunscreens, tanning lotions
- Astringents, exfoliants
- Cosmetics that contain aloe, camphor, castor oil, witch hazel, ginseng, or any salicylate
- Lipsticks with aloe, camphor, or castor oil
- Shampoos, conditioners, or hair sprays with plant derivatives, including herbs, lavender, almond, cucumber, and others
- Dandruff shampoos
- Bubble baths and lotions
- Deodorants with castor oil
- Shaving creams with aloe, mint, or mentholatum
- Razors with aloe strips
- Mint, wintergreen mouthwashes and toothpastes, and any mouthwash with salicylate

Dr. St. Amand cautions that his program is "not for the weak of courage." As reversal worsens symptoms, the first two to four months can be more debilitating than the preexisting fibromyalgia, and according to Dr. St. Amand, "It takes confidence and strength to get through this early phase."

Low-Carbohydrate Diet

A low-carbohydrate diet can also help a common symptom of CFS and fibromyalgia, hypoglycemia. Dr. R. Paul St. Amand, who created the "guaifenisin protocol," also created the term "fibroglycemia," for hypoglycemia in people with fibromyalgia. According to Dr. St. Amand, eliminating the following foods can prevent fluctuations in blood sugar and help minimize fatigue:

All alcohol, dried fruits, fruit juice, baked beans, refried beans, lima beans, barley, black-eyed peas (cowpeas), lentils, garbanzos, rice, bananas, pastas (all types), flour tortillas as in burritos, tamales, corn, potatoes, and sweets of any kind— including dextrose, glucose, hexitol, maltose, sucrose, honey, fructose, corn syrup, or starch.

Is It Worth It?

Dr. St. Amand and some of the patients who have followed his program, or who are participating in his online support groups, are strong proponents of the guaifenesin protocol. But there is no research proving that the protocol works. The evidence and support for its success is, to date, anecdotal. There was one double-blind, placebo-controlled study of guaifenesin, conducted in 1995 by Robert Bennett, M.D., and researchers at the University of Oregon. In this study, time-released guaifenesin at 600 mg was given twice a day to twenty women with fibromyalgia. The results showed that the guaifenesin was no more effective at relieving fibromyalgia symptoms than the placebo.

Dr. St. Amand feels that this study was flawed, however, and believes that the outcome was due to some patients being blocked by use of salicylates, as well as some patients being hypoglycemic, and also the dosage being insufficient for some patients. He challenges the results, claiming that the protocol is being used by hundreds of doctors to great success.

The Musculoskeletal Connection

The human body is an energy system which is never a complete
structure; never static; is in perpetual inner self-construction and
self-destruction; we destroy in order to make it new.
—NORMAN O. BROWN

There are a variety of musculoskeletal issues that may have a role
in the development of CFS and, particularly, fibromyalgia.

■ Post-Traumatic Fibromyalgia

One area of great interest is the study of post-traumatic fibromyalgia. This refers to the theory that an accident or injury that causes
even mild or moderate trauma to the brain may trigger fibromyalgia. Theoretically, post-traumatic fibromyalgia can result from a
single episode of trauma (such as a car accident) or a series of
injuries over time.

What may be happening is that an injury releases pain-
inducing chemicals into the injured area, but in fibromyalgia,
instead of healing and returning to normal, the release of pain-
stimulating chemicals continues, and even affects other areas of

the body, which then react with more pain signals, causing a cascading effect.

While it's controversial, neck injury, and in particular whiplash, appears to be the area most linked to development of fibromyalgia. One Swiss study looked at the degree of central nervous system sensitization among patients with whiplash, fibromyalgia, and healthy controls. Only the fibromyalgia and whiplash patients showed evidence of increased sensitization.

Another ongoing study in Seattle is looking at onset of fibromyalgia after whiplash. Ultimately, the target is to study 400 whiplash patients. Among the people studied to date, 20 percent have developed widespread pain and 80 percent met the tender-point criteria for a diagnosis of fibromyalgia.

One study in Israel found that there is a tenfold increase in the risk of developing fibromyalgia within a year of neck injury. A follow-up to the Israeli study looked at 78 patients with neck injury three years after the original study. Twenty of the original 22 patients who developed fibromyalgia after neck injury were also reevaluated. What the researchers discovered was that 60 percent percent of the twenty patients who had FMS in 1996 still had it after three years. All of the women who had been diagnosed still met fibromyalgia criteria, but only 1 of the 9 men still did. And among the patients who did not have fibromyalgia after one year, only 1 of 58 patients went on to develop the condition after three years. Most patients reported improved quality of life, with less tenderness, and all had remained employed. These findings led researchers to conclude that post-traumatic fibromyalgia outcomes were potentially better for men than women, and that if a patient does not develop fibromyalgia within a year, the likelihood is very small that they will develop it later.

■ Treatments

"EEG-Slowing" Treatment Protocol

One expert in traumatic brain injury, Mary Lee Esty, Ph.D., has found that in fibromyalgia patients "EEG slowing" occurs, where the brain's most powerful electrical activity is found in the slowest brain waves—i.e., delta, theta, and alpha waves. The theory is that trauma, viruses, severe stress, or even rape or abuse can damage brain cells, which causes the brain to shift to slower waves as a protective mechanism.

EEG slowing can be diagnosed and treated using the electroencephalogram (EEG) brain-mapping technique and processing known as SyNAPs, or synergistic neurotherapy adjustment process. Areas of brain wave dysfunction receive rhythmic electrical stimulation, which redirects power from slower to faster waves, enabling more appropriate handling of pain signals in the brain. This process, combined with neuromuscular reeducation techniques, has had promising results.

Physical Therapy

There are many physical therapy treatment options for CFS and fibromyalgia patients. Physical therapy can provide relief from some symptoms, and over time help minimize pain responses.

Ultrasound. Ultrasound gives off high-frequency sound waves that can direct heat deep into soft tissues, promoting circulation, relaxing muscles, reducing pain, and helping to decrease inflammation.

Electrical stimulation. This technique involves the use of electrodes to stimulate a particular muscle area, forcing it to contract and relax. The process helps with healing, and reduces swelling and pain.

Heat. A common physical therapy technique, heat—in the form of heating pads, moist heat, warm baths, paraffin dips, and hot showers, among others—can help reduce stiffness, increase circulation, and reduce pain. Heat is particularly helpful for back pain. Warm, moist heat typically helps relieve myofascial/muscle pain.

Cold. Application of cold, in the form of ice or cold packs, slows down nerve impulses and reduces the temperature below the skin, reducing inflammation and decreasing pain. Cold typically relieves pain from entrapped nerves.

Hands-on. These therapies, which include spray and stretch, osteopathic manipulation, manual healing/bodywork, and trigger point therapy/myofascial release, can help with joint mobility, range of motion, increased circulation, and pain reduction.

Treating Trigger Points

For patients who have pain in identifiable trigger points, there are a variety of therapies that may be helpful.

Spray and stretch. The spray-and-stretch technique is particularly popular with physical therapists treating fibromyalgia patients. It involves passively stretching a particular muscle while applying a spray coolant on the skin. The coldness of the spray produces a temporary anesthesia, allowing for a greater stretch with less pain. This is thought to deactivate trigger points, relieve muscle spasm, and reduce referred pain. After stretch-and-spray therapy, moist heat is usually applied for ten to twenty minutes, followed by some range-of-motion work to help maintain the results.

Trigger point therapy. This involves putting pressure on the trigger points, for example, using finger or elbow, to deactivate a painful trigger point. A trained practitioner of trigger point or myofascial release therapy must perform this type of therapy.

Cranial electrotherapy stimulation. One promising trigger point treatment is cranial electrotherapy stimulation, or CES. In CES electrodes are clipped to the ear lobes and low-level electrical stimulation currents then pass across the head. One double-blind, peer-reviewed study of CES showed a 28 percent improvement in tender point scores and a 27 percent improvement in self-reported pain levels. One particularly promising result was that those patients reporting poor quality of sleep dropped from 60 percent to only 5 percent after treatment.

Injection Therapy

This type of treatment involves injections into painful points, or trigger points. There are several different ways this can be approached.

Trigger point injections. These are injections of medication directly into the trigger point, with the goal of deactivating the point. This is usually done with an anesthetic such as procaine (Novocain) or lidocaine (Xylocaine). (Note: Corticosteroids such as cortisone are not used or recommended for injection since they have no benefit in trigger point therapy.) "Dry needling" is a form of trigger point injection that doesn't include any anesthetic. These can sometimes be more painful, however. Ultimately, the object is to deactivate the trigger point to the extent that the muscle can be stretched and reconditioned back to a more normal state.

Botulinum toxin type A. Known as Botox or Myobloc, this drug is one cutting-edge treatment for some of the pain associated with fibromyalgia. Some patients have reported several months of relief in their tender points after Botox injections. The effects may take about a week to be felt, and the greatest amount of relief usually is felt within four weeks of receiving the injection. Botox can be costly, running as much as $400 per shot. Another study showed that 30 to 40 percent of the patients receiving Botox injections reported significant improvement in their pain and overall functioning. Botox injections can be performed with electromyograph machine (EMG) guidance to help specifically identify the trigger point.

Ketamine. Ketamine injections are considered particularly promising. At lower levels, ketamine blocks the NMDA (N-methyl-D-aspartate) receptors. At high doses ketamine is an anesthetic. A French study looked at the effectiveness of subcutaneous ketamine for fibromyalgia pain. Treatment was using an infusion pump similar to that used by diabetics. Seventy-eight percent of the patients reported significant improvement in pain scores, and 45 percent still reported some improvement as long as six months later.

Other forms of injectable pain relief that are less frequently used include facet block, which injects pain relief into the facet joints around the vertebrae from the base of the skull to the tailbone, which are a common source of pain. Epidurals are occasionally done, injecting pain relievers into the epidural lining. And peripheral nerve blocks combine an anesthetic and steroid and are used for pain triggered by nerve problems such as carpal tunnel syndrome, or a trapped nerve.

Osteopathic Manipulation

Osteopathic manipulation works with the musculoskeletal system to treat illness, which in osteopathic theory, can result from imbalances and misalignment in the body's structure. As part of their broader family practice functions, many osteopathic physicians rely on this osteopathic manipulation as a form of treatment. Some M.D. practitioners also have been trained in osteopathic manipulation and can provide this sort of therapy.

There is clear research supporting the use of osteopathic manipulation and techniques for musculoskeletal and nonmusculoskeletal problems. Osteopathic manipulation is particularly useful in terms of muscular and joint pain relief, and for problems such as carpal tunnel syndrome or chronic sinusitis. Personally, I've found osteopathic manipulation to be most useful in dealing with various muscle trauma and joint pain, such as a case of whiplash I had after being rear-ended in my car. The manipulation enabled the use of far fewer painkillers and muscle relaxants, and speeded up the healing process.

If you want to find an osteopath, you'll definitely need someone who has a D.O. degree from a four-year medical college accredited by the American Association of Colleges of Osteopathic Medicine.

Manual Healing/Bodywork

Manual healing and bodywork can be particularly helpful for CFS and fibromyalgia patients. This is a broad category that focuses on the use of touch to heal the body. Massage and manipulation are among the oldest methods of health care. In bodywork, manual techniques, using hands, arms, elbows, and sometimes even feet, apply various types of pressure to affect the muscles, bones, joints, circulation, and other body systems.

There are so many different forms of massage, manual healing and movement therapy, that it's hard even to list them all. Swedish massage, trigger point massage (myotherapy, neuromuscular massage therapy), Rolfing, Trager, Alexander technique, Feldenkrais, myofascial release technique, and other realignment therapies concentrate on the soft tissue surrounding the bones. Practitioners of reflexology and acupressure stimulate points so as to clear energy pathways that appear to be blocked. And there are many kinds of energy work, such as Reiki and therapeutic touch, in which the therapist is a conduit for healing energy that is directed to the patient through the therapist's hands, sometimes without actually touching the client.

Any type of bodywork can be useful, and it depends on your body and your own preferences. It's most important to find a good therapist with whom you are comfortable. Before choosing a therapist, talk with several about their work so you can get a feel for whether you think you can work with them. A therapist should be willing to give you at least some telephone time, but you might want to pay for a brief office consult if you have many questions.

Bodywork can be quite helpful for CFS and fibromyalgia, particularly if the therapist is familiar with the conditions and is able to offer a combination of techniques. Medical studies have found various forms of massage and physical therapy to be effective in dealing with pain, depression, energy, insomnia, and inflammation, among other things. Some myofascial and myotherapy experts have had particular success working with the fibromyalgia and chronic fatigue symptoms.

There are different licensing and accreditation requirements for each type of bodywork. Many specialty areas such as Rolfing and Feldenkrais offer separate certification. Some states and areas license massage therapists. The main certification to look for, however, is N.C.T.M.B., which is granted by the National Certification Board for Therapeutic Massage & Bodywork after completion of five hundred hours of training and passage of an exam.

Acupuncture

One way acupuncture works is by helping change the body's pain perceptions and releasing endorphins, the body's natural painkillers.

The impact of acupuncture on CFS has not been extensively studied. But even though there haven't been large-scale clinical trials, there is fairly strong evidence that acupuncture can be effective in treating fibromyalgia symptoms.

In one study of 60 fibromyalgia patients, all patients received amitriptyline for pain and at bedtime. One group of 20 also had a weekly thirty-minute acupuncture session; a second group of 20 had a thirty-minute weekly mock acupuncture session, with treatment in areas not believed to have any effect on pain. Patients who received real acupuncture were the only ones to show statistically significant improvement in measurement of pain, depression and mental health, and results were seen within a month, and lasted as long as sixteen weeks.

A Swiss study of 70 patients found that 75 percent showed improvement in their disease with acupuncture treatments. And researchers at the Federal University of São Paulo, Brazil, have done a study showing that acupuncture can help relieve symptoms such as pain and depression in fibromyalgia.

■ Exercise

Exercise for Fibromyalgia

Exercise is an area of contention for both CFS and fibromyalgia patients. For a percentage of CFS and fibromyalgia patients, exercise may be impossible, or when attempted may trigger painful and debilitating relapses that require days or more of recovery.

It's important to look at the issues around exercise separately.

First, many practitioners believe that exercise—but only to tolerance—is an important part of fibromyalgia treatment and recovery. Exercise has many important effects in the body:

• Increases serotonin levels
• Helps with dysautonomia symptoms
• Helps improve flexibility and reduce muscle tension
• Increases time spent in deep sleep

In one study reported in the journal *Arthritis Care & Research*, researchers stated that patients with fibromyalgia found exercise more effective at alleviating symptoms than medication or other alternative treatments. A third of the patients reported that they had approximately a 30 percent improvement in pain symptoms.

A British study found that exercise could significantly ease pain in patients with fibromyalgia. The study looked at 136 fibromyalgia patients who were assigned to either aerobic exercise or a relaxation and flexibility exercise program. Tender points and other symptoms were assessed at the onset. After three months, 24 of the 69 in the aerobic exercise group rated themselves as "much or very much better," compared to 12 of 67 of the patients in the relaxation and flexibility group. After a year, 26 of the patients in the exercise group had continued improvements, compared to 15 in the relaxation group. The exercise group also had greater reductions in tender point counts and symptoms. After a year, fewer patients in the aerobic exercise group met the criteria for fibromyalgia than the other group, showing that exercise was effective in helping to reverse their fibromyalgia.

What "exercising to tolerance" means is that the exercise should take the fibromyalgia into consideration, but not be avoided or minimized entirely. Stretching and exercise should be as strenuous as possible without causing any pain during the activity, and without triggering postexercise fatigue, pain, or other relapsing symptoms.

An exercise should be individualized and customized. If at all possible, work with a rehabilitative trainer or take a physical therapy-oriented exercise class—such as warm-water aerobics for arthritis—at the start of your exercise efforts.

Many experts agree that the optimal exercise program for fibromyalgia should include

- Strengthening exercises
- Passive stretching
- Postural exercises
- Low-impact aerobic exercise (i.e., cycling, swimming, walking
- Starting with just a few minutes a session, gradually increasing up to three sessions a week of exercise, approximately forty minutes per session

- Reaching a pulse rate of 85 percent of the target heart rate for age

Exercise for CFS

Practitioners do advise exercise for CFS patients, especially to prevent deconditioning, and believe that all but the most incapacitated should do some sort of physical exercise, even if it's just a few minutes a day. But patients should not have worsening of symptoms after exercise.

The key issue is what to do, how much, and when to stop, so that the activity contributes to well-being rather than becoming debilitating or worsening fatigue.

Gina is a patient who has modified exercise to fit her condition:

I have tried many times to do aerobic exercises, but usually end up hurting too much to continue. I find that walking is my best exercise, and doing steps or jumping around is not helpful. Swimming in warm water is good, but too cold water makes me too tense to relax.

Modest regular exercise to avoid deconditioning is important. A knowledgeable health-care provider or physical therapist should supervise the program of exercise and/or the exercise itself. Such supervision is especially important for severely compromised patients.

Even some of those with debilitating CFS are able to do some simple exercise. Some of the least-taxing exercises that can still provide benefit include

- Chair exercises
- Tai chi
- Simple walking

- Use of light hand weights
- Limbering/stretching
- Basic Pilates (Pilates is a method of exercise and movement designed to stretch, strengthen, and balance the body especially the core area of the abdomen and lower back.)

Graded Exercise for CFS

The CFS/ME Working Group in Britain issued a controversial study in 2002 outlining strategies for helping with the condition. One of their primary recommendations is what's called "graded exercise," which is a form of structured and supervised exercise that focuses on slow and gradual increases in aerobic activity. There is a great deal of controversy over making this a key recommendation because the study had a one-third dropout rate, and excluded people who weren't able to go to outpatient clinics. Basically, those who were unable to exercise weren't counted in the overall survey total, so results are thought to be skewed. Among the 1,214 severely affected people studied, 610 believed graded exercise made their condition worse, 417 found it helpful, and 187 reported no change.

Pacing

Another of Britain's CFS/ME Working Group three key recommendations for CFS is what's called "pacing." Pacing is a systematic way of balancing rest and activity so as to avoid activities that worsen symptoms, and includes resting during periods of improvement.

Often patients who feel better will attempt to do too much on days when they have more energy. That excess activity can trigger a setback, and the person requires days to recuperate. The theory is that a person with CFS or fibromyalgia may have only a finite amount of energy, and must live within that energy budget. Some practitioners believe that patients should not spend more than 70 percent or 80 percent of their perceived energy.

The issue of pacing is controversial, since some doctors believe that pacing may perpetuate the illness. Patients and organizations support pacing, however, and 89 percent in one survey of 2,000 patients claimed to find the practice of pacing helpful.

Some pacing tips:

• Divide projects into smaller tasks, and only do a small amount at a time, with rests in between. For example, it might be easier to read a few pages and go back to a book later rather than read a chapter straight through.

• Use less energy during activities—for example, sit when ironing.

• Be organized so you do not spend valuable energy going up and down stairs or around your house looking for lost or misplaced items.

• If finances permit, hire help for things like housecleaning and yardwork, and save your energy for activities you enjoy most.

• Alternate activity and rest, and alternate mental and physical activities.

Yoga, Tai Chi, Pilates, Qigong

Some of the stretching and balance-oriented exercises such as yoga, tai chi, and Pilates are ideal for CFS and fibromyalgia patients because they involve slow, deliberate, nonimpact movements. The spirit of both practices is noncompetitive, and they emphasize the ability to perform the movements slowly, properly, carefully, with mindfulness and awareness. As exercises that also have mind–body aspects, they also help with mood and depression.

YOGA   Yoga is not just standing on your head or sitting in the lotus position. It's an ancient science and art that seeks to balance the body, mind, and spirit internally and externally. Yoga's physical exercises, breathing exercises, and meditation techniques help achieve that union and balance. Some forms of yoga, such as the "Yoga in Daily Life" approach popular in the U.S., are ideal for rehabilitative purposes, since they are low-stress forms of yoga that are easily adapted to those who are not in optimal condition. Yoga's many benefits are proven. For example, certain forms of yoga have been found to have a strong antidepressant effect. Yoga also has been found to improve lung function and breathing. And yoga can help with various neuropathies, dysautonomia, and other problems.

CFS researcher and professor of family medicine Arthur Hartz, M.D., Ph.D., along with his associate Suzanne Bentler conducted a study more than five years ago looking at 150 patients with CFS and evaluating the various treatments they were using. Two years later, they reevaluated the study subjects, determining who had reported improvement in symptoms, and found, surprisingly, that yoga apparently helped patients more than any other treatment approach.

The inverted poses seem to have particular benefit for CFS patients. Dr. Hartz feels that the inversions may be helping to address the neurally mediated hypotension—where blood pressure drops while standing.

Some of the poses found most useful include

- The supported Ardha-Halasana (half-plow pose)
- Salamba sirsasana I (supported headstand)
- Salamba Sarvangasana (supported shoulder stand)
- Supported Savasana (corpse pose)
- Viparita Karani (legs-up-on-the-wall pose)

Joyce is a big fan of yoga to help with her symptoms:

The non-medical thing that I do that helps me is yoga—Iyengar form—which is more slow moving and more precise and demanding than most Hatha Yoga. I am careful to hold poses only as long as I am comfortable so that I will not get worse afterwards. Yoga helps the body be in better alignment, helps stretch muscles that are tight, and helps strengthen muscles. When I consistently practice yoga I experience less pain and feel better. I have more energy. I gradually become stronger.

TAI CHI   Tai chi, also known as tai chi chuan, is a form of exercise that originated in China. Tai chi coordinates movements of the body with the mind and breathing, and emphasizes flexibility, balance, and serenity of both mind and body. In one study, it was found that people who practiced tai chi had improved balance, flexibility, and cardiovascular fitness when compared to sedentary Parkinson's patients. Other studies have shown that tai chi can improve balance in older practitioners. A 1997 study at Atlanta's Emory University found that a fifteen-week modified tai chi program significantly reduced falls in a group of older seniors.

Patients who practice tai chi on a regular basis report that they are sleeping better, have improved energy levels, and have an improved sense of balance. Some patients have enjoyed a reduction in their rate of falling or stumbling, and one patient stopped using her cane and walker after three months of practicing tai chi.

THE PILATES METHOD   The Pilates Method is an exercise system that focuses on improving flexibility and strength for the total body by focusing on strengthening the "powerhouse"—the abdomen, lower back, and buttocks—so that the rest of the body is supported. Pilates is recommended by physical therapists, chiropractors, and orthopedists, and is frequently part of rehabilitative exercise and physical therapy programs. Pilates can be performed at a studio or gym that has the Pilates apparatus, or various Pilates exercises can be performed on the floor in what's known as Pilates Matwork.

When regularly practiced, Pilates can increase lung capacity and circulation; increase flexibility in the back; reduce pain in back, neck, and shoulders; and reduce depression. Pilates is considered as an effective method of movement reeducation and form of physical therapy and rehabilitation for people with neurological, chronic pain, and orthopedic conditions.

QIGONG *Qi* means "energy," and *gong* means "skill," and qigong is the Chinese self-healing art that combines posture, gentle movement, breathing techniques, concentration, and meditation to attract energy and improve health. Qigong is not particularly strenuous, but is energizing, and may be a good choice for CFS and fibromyalgia patients who don't have energy for more rigorous exercise.

CHOOSING WHAT'S BEST FOR YOU Yoga, tai chi, Pilates, and qigong classes are increasingly available at community centers, rehabilitation centers, senior centers, fitness centers, and many other locations. Personal trainers and some physical therapists can also provide training and direction in these areas.

Your selection of the right class and trainer is particularly important. Many fibromyalgia and CFS patients could take a gentle, beginner's yoga class, but might require some adaptation or modification to accommodate limitations. Some practitioners actually teach yoga classes for people with physical disabilities featuring only poses that can be done in a chair or lying down. There are many styles and classes of yoga, so be careful before signing up for any classes or yoga centers. Yoga has become trendy, and there are some forms of yoga that are amazingly rigorous and inappropriate for a CFS or fibromyalgia patient. Pilates, another trendy entry into the exercise arena, depends on the instructor. Some classes are more rehabilitative in nature, and others are more rigorous. Tai chi and qi gong are usually gentle, and shouldn't be a problem at any fitness level.

Most important, a CFS or fibromyalgia patient considering an exercise class or trainer should consider talking to the class leader or trainer to discuss the style of class or exercise and your own limitations. Do they have chairs, pillows, and props available, and will they incorporate them into the class for those who have difficulty balancing, standing, reaching, or sitting on the floor? Ask how challenging the regimen will be for someone who doesn't have as much strength or flexibility. How much practice will be expected between sessions in order for you to keep up? Consider sitting in on a class to see whether it's to your liking.

◼ Chiari Malformation

There is a line of research that believes that some cases of CFS and fibromyalgia may result from what's known as a Chiari malformation, also called Arnold-Chiari malformation. In Chiari malformation, the cerebellar "tonsils"—a portion of the brain that is shaped like the tonsils in the throat—extend several millimeters down through an opening in the base of the skull. This is the opening that the spinal cord passes through on its way to attaching to the brain. With a Chiari malformation, the cerebellar tonsils extend into that opening, putting pressure on and compressing both the brain stem and spinal cord.

A perhaps lesser known but more common condition is cervical stenosis, where the spinal canal is actually too narrow for the spinal cord, also causing pressure and compression on the brain stem and spinal cord.

While some of these problems are congenital, some may be due to traumatic injury or worsened by an injury such as whiplash. Symptoms may present themselves suddenly or slowly over time.

Chiari malformation/spinal cord compression can cause a variety of symptoms, some of the most common being

- Headache in the back of the head
- Headache that radiates behind the eyes and into the neck and shoulders
- Disordered eye movements, vision changes
- Dysautonomia symptoms (dizziness, orthostatic intolerance, neurally mediated hypotension)
- Muscle weakness
- Unsteadiness when walking
- Cold, numbness, and tingling in the extremities
- Buzzing or ringing in the ears, or hearing loss
- Difficulty speaking, swallowing

Diagnosis

If you're interested in pursuing Chiari diagnosis and treatment, you'll need to see a neurologist or neurosurgeon with experience in treating Chiari malformations. In fact, consider seeing only one of the few physicians in the country who are considered the experts in diagnosis and treatment of Chiari malformation, some of whom are listed in the Resources section.

Diagnosis should include high-level MRIs, detailed neurological testing, and evaluation to rule out cervical spinal stenosis, because decompression surgery for a Chiari malformation can actually worsen cervical stenosis symptoms.

Treatment

The treatment for Chiari malformation is surgery to remove some bone in the skull and or vertebrae, making additional space for the brain stem and spinal cord and eliminating the compression.

Chiari surgery is quite controversial. Some surgeons disagree as to whether or not to perform a craniectomy, removing more skull to create space, versus removing some of the dura, the membrane covering the brain.

There is also controversy over the results. Some patients report success, claiming, for example, that their CFS is "cured" or that fibromyalgia trigger points have completely disappeared. Others, however, have complained that their symptoms have worsened after surgery. And there is no way to anticipate who will benefit from this type of surgery.

One patient, Gretchen, described her experience with Chiari surgery:

Unfortunately, the surgery did not alleviate most of my symptoms. I did get relief of my postural orthostatic tachycardia syndrome (POTS), however. When speaking with my doctor in follow up appointments, he said that in some cases, even though the MRIs might look the same between patients, sometimes surgery doesn't help, and I was one of those cases. There was nothing further he knew to do.

13

Why get up, why get up
How can I get up, why should I get up
This whole world's gone crazy
Think I've seen enough
I'm gonna sleep forever, why get up
—THE FABULOUS THUNDERBIRDS
(B. Carter/R. Ellsworth)

■ Sleep Dysfunction

Some researchers believe that CFS and fibromyalgia may be, at their core, primarily sleep disorders. Others believe that sleep disruptions are important components in CFS and fibromyalgia. But all practitioners agree that getting sufficient high-quality sleep is probably one of the most basic, most critical elements in maintaining a healthy, strong immune system.

During typical sleep, every ninety minutes you move from light alpha sleep (stage 1) into progressively deeper sleep, beta (stage 2) and gamma (stage 3), until you reach delta sleep (stage 4), the most refreshing and restorative stage of sleep. Light alpha sleep is also known as REM (rapid eye movement) sleep, when you have dreams. Stages 2, 3, and 4 are non-REM sleep.

Unfortunately, one of the most common symptoms of both CFS and fibromyalgia is the disruption of sleep. One survey of more than 1,000 CFS and fibromyalgia patients found that less than 1 percent had sleep disturbances prior to developing their illness, but 90 percent developed sleep disruptions.

Some studies have shown that as many as half of all fibromyalgia patients have disturbed stage 4 delta sleep.

There are so many ways that sleep problems can manifest themselves:

- Insomnia
- Difficulty falling asleep
- Frequent waking
- Difficulty falling asleep after waking
- Frequent waking to urinate
- Failure to reach deep, stage 4 sleep
- Unrefreshing sleep
- Sleep apnea (episodes where breathing stops longer than normal), which occurs in around 25 percent of CFS and fibromyalgia patients
- Sleep myoclonus, nighttime muscle contractions, twitching, and restless leg syndrome) estimated to affect 16 percent of patients
- Bruxism (grinding of teeth) affects between 10 and 15 percent of patients

Restorative sleep—also known as stage 4, or delta, sleep—is the most crucial stage of sleep. It is during this stage that the body recovers energy and repairs muscle tissue. Without delta sleep, a person might sleep eight hours yet wake feeling unrefreshed.

If you don't get enough sleep, particularly stage 4 delta sleep, a number of things can happen to your immune system:

- Your level of natural killer (NK) cells can drop.
- Your level of growth hormone may become low. Since 80 percent of growth hormone is produced during delta sleep, insufficient delta sleep can result in growth hormone deficiencies, which can contribute to muscular pain and degeneration.
- You can develop fatigue, aching muscles, and trigger point tenderness. One study showed that interrupting delta sleep for three nights in a row caused test subjects to develop these symptoms.
- You may develop brain fog.

Diagnosing a sleep disorder can be done through a formal sleep study. Some practitioners recommend a less expensive, simpler process: Set up a video camera to tape your sleeping at night, so you and your practitioner can observe your sleep behaviors.

Sleep Hygiene

Sleep hygiene, a term to describe the environment and practices surrounding your sleep, is often the first place to start addressing sleep dysfunction. Here are some tips on proper sleep hygiene:

- Don't take afternoon naps if at all possible, or limit naps to no more than an hour.
- Avoid stimulants/caffeine/alcohol, especially four hours before bedtime. Since caffeine builds up throughout the day, you may want to avoid caffeine after lunch.
- Avoid late-night snacks. If you must eat something before bed, try a small snack rich in carbohydrates. Milk products, in particular, are rich in tryptophan, which can help with sleep. So consider a piece of low-fat cheese, or a snack with a small glass of milk.
- Eat well and maintain a balanced diet.
- Maintain a steady sleep pattern. Don't go to sleep at 2 a.m. one day only to hit the hay at 7 p.m. the next. This goes for waking up, too.

- Exercise regularly, but not right before bedtime. Try to stay active even if you are bored, tired, or in pain.
- Limit stress and physical stimulants in the bedroom. That means no television in the bedroom or stacks of undone work.
- Don't eat dinner late in the evening. Digestion requires energy and can make you less able to sleep.
- Don't watch television late into the evening.
- Try mindfulness or meditative techniques, including breathing, prayer, or guided imagery.
- Minimize noise and light by using earplugs or a white-noise machine, eyeshades, window shades, or light-blocking curtains.
- Avoid temperature extremes, and use an electric blanket or air conditioner as needed.
- Don't spend time in bed except for sleeping or sex. Otherwise you will associate bed with eating, work, reading, television, and other awake activities.
- Give yourself an hour to unwind before bed, creating a routine for going to sleep.
- Get morning light therapy: As soon as you wake up, open blinds, turn on lights, and get as much light as you can.

Specialty Bedding

Some of the specialty beds that may be of help include flotation beds such as waterbeds, airbeds, latex resilient-foam beds, visco-elastic foam beds, adjustable beds, and combination beds that include various technologies.

Some people find it helpful to have a special mattress topper that relieves the pressure points when they are sleeping. Some patients report that foam pads—particularly the "egg crate" style—help.

For optimal comfort, however, patients frequently prefer a wool mattress underquilt or topper. One in particular that is very popular with CFS and fibromyalgia patients is the Cuddle Ewe underquilt, which is filled with layers of thick, natural wool batting.

Placed between the mattress and bottom sheet, the Cuddle Ewe underquilt supports and distributes body weight and manages temperature. A professor of medicine at the University of Texas Health Science Center's Division of Clinical Immunology studied the Cuddle Ewe and reported that "Cuddle Ewe underquilts significantly improve the quality and quantity of sleep for people with fibromyalgia syndrome."

Note from Mary: I have a Cuddle Ewe, and I love it. It definitely keeps you warmer in winter and cooler in summer. I feel like it cradles me, and is easy on the tender points and sore spots. I've gotten so accustomed to it that it's hard to sleep away from my own bed!

Nonprescription Sleep Aids

• Over-the-counter drugs, such as those containing diphenhydramine (Benadryl, Tylenol PM, ExcedrinPM), that are not habit-forming. Some experts disagree, saying that because these products do not induce deep sleep, they aren't of help to people with FMS.

• Melatonin, particularly helpful if your body clock is off-kilter and you're finding yourself unable to go to sleep until early in the morning. Take 1 mg to 3 mg if you are under the age of fifty, up to 6 mg over fifty, at bedtime, but if you wake up groggy, it may be too much—cut the dose back.

• Magnesium and/or calcium.

• Doxylamine (Unisom)—(an antihistamine). For sleep: 25 mg at night.

• 5-HTP (5-hydroxytryptophan): 100 to 400 mg at night. Naturally stimulates serotonin.

Herbal Treatments

Some of the herbs that have been reported to help with sleep include valerian root, passionflower, and kava kava.

After trying a variety of herbal supplements, CFS/fibromyalgia practitioner Jacob Teitelbaum, M.D., formulated a special herbal combination supplement called Revitalizing Sleep Formula that contains the exact combination of ingredients he has found most effective in facilitating stage 4 sleep without morning grogginess. The supplement is available at most health food and vitamin stores, and includes

- Valerian (*Valeriana officinalis*) root extract
- Passionflower (*Passiflora incarnata*) leaf flower extract
- L-theanine
- Hops (*Humulus lupulus*) flower extract
- Wild lettuce (*Lactuca virosa*) leaf extract
- Jamaican dogwood (*Piscidia piscipula*) root extract

Prescription Sleep Aids

- **Tricyclic antidepressants.** Antidepressants can help to relieve pain and to increase serotonin levels, both functions that can facilitate improved sleep. Frequently prescribed for sleep disturbances and pain in CFS and fibromyalgia are low doses of tricyclic antidepressants, including doxepin (Adapin, Sinequan), amitriptyline (Elavil, Etrafon, Limbitrol, Triavil), desipramine (Norpramin), and nortriptyline (Pamelor). These drugs may provide long-term benefit for improving sleep.

- **Other antidepressants.** Other antidepressants that may be prescribed include sertraline (Zoloft), venlafaxine (Effexor), fluvoxamine (Luvox), fluoxetine (Prozac), paroxetine (Paxil), and mirtazapine (Remeron). Typically, it can take six weeks of using the antidepressant before it has any impact on sleep.

- **Trazodone (Desyrel).** This is a frequently prescribed antidepressant for sleep problems, aiding with stage 3 and 4 sleep. It's particularly helpful for those who wake up every hour, or wake up and then can't go back to sleep.

- **Reboxetine (Edronax, Vestra).** This is a relatively new antidepressant that seems to be particularly helpful for patients who have pain and lethargy, which are common in CFS and fibromyalgia. One study found a significant reduction in fibromyalgia pain in approximately a third of participants. Some of the patients also reported a feeling of increased energy, which was a positive effect for most patients.

- **Antianxiety drugs/muscle relaxants/benzodiazepines.** These are drugs that can help improve sleep, relax muscles, and modulate brain and brain receptor sensitivity. The most frequently recommended drug in CFS and fibromyalgia is clonazepam (Klonopin), a long-acting benzodiazepine. Klonopin also can help with myoclonus and restless leg syndrome. Others include lorazepam (Ativan) and alprazolam (Xanax). Habit-forming potential may be a concern with these drugs.

- **Hypnotics.** The hypnotic drugs include zolpidem (Ambien), triazolam (Halcion), temazepam (Restoril), flurazepam (Dalmane), quazepam (Doral), and estazolam (ProSom). Habit-forming potential may be a concern with these drugs. The drug zaleplon (Sonata) is a new sleep drug that is considered non–habit-forming, and may be a better option than the potentially habit-forming hypnotics.

Dr. Teitelbaum believes that you can and should, under the careful direction of your practitioner, take as many different prescription and herbal treatments as you need until you are getting seven to eight hours of sleep without waking, and are waking refreshed.

■ Biopsychosocial/Cognitive

Some two thousand years ago, the philosopher Epictetus said "The thing that upsets people is not what happens but what they think it means."

This is the crux of the idea behind the "biopsychosocial" and cognitive part of CFS and fibromyalgia. Biopsychosociology is a fancy way of saying that your health and conditions, and the possibility for improvement, are affected by and in some cases linked to your beliefs, your coping styles, and your behaviors.

To say that CFS and fibromyalgia have a biopsychosocial component is to say your thoughts, beliefs, attitudes, and biases influence your emotions, and the intensity of your emotions, particularly as related to your disease.

Don't misunderstand the concept that beliefs, coping, and behavior are linked to your health. This is *not* suggesting in any way that CFS or fibromyalgia are psychosomatic, brought on by emotional problems, or a figment of your imagination. Because they are most definitely not. And you should not put up with any suggestion otherwise—whether from health-care practitioner, family member, or friend.

But it is a fact that your behavior and how you cope with your condition will have an impact on how you feel and your long-term efforts to feel and live well.

As an example, imagine the phone rings at 4 a.m. How would you feel? Your immediate reaction might be that your heart starts pounding and your mouth goes dry as you imagine that there's terrible news on the other end of the line. But suppose you suddenly remember that your spouse is traveling abroad, where it's actually late morning. You pick up the phone, and it's your spouse, who has forgotten the time difference and is just checking in to say hello. How do you feel now? You probably don't feel frightened or anxious. You might be annoyed by the middle-of-the-night wake-up! This is all to illustrate that how you are feeling is somewhat determined by what you think. In this example, your initial feelings of fear were totally based on how you were interpreting a middle-of-the-night phone call.

Cognitive therapy is designed to help you learn to think constructively and more realistically about many day-to-day events and life issues that can otherwise cause you stress. Cognitive therapy helps you avoid a tendency to think negatively about various happenings. Many practitioners believe that cognitive therapy is an essential part of managing the condition for many patients. You should not feel that a suggestion of cognitive therapy is the practitioner saying that the condition is "in your head." Rather cognitive therapy can be an effective part of your overall treatment approach, and can complement the other approaches that are part of your plan.

In one study, patients who participated in a fibromyalgia rehabilitation program that relied on cognitive therapy approaches had significant clinical benefits in all ways, except for actual physical function. In Canada, a ten-week program was developed for fibromyalgia patients. The program featured educational programs, group support, training in coping skills, water exercise, goal setting and maintaining a diary of daily activity. A total of 395 fibromyalgia patients were analyzed, and very significant improvements were seen in terms of symptoms and functioning among most of the patients. Another study looked at 145 patients with fibromyalgia who were all given standard treatment for the condition, including antidepressants, pain-relievers, and instructions about exercise. Half of the patients also received six sessions of cognitive behavioral therapy conducted over four weeks. The patients who went through the therapy were evaluated a year later, and the researchers found that 25 percent of patients experienced a significant increase in physical functioning after the treatment versus improvement in only 12 percent of patients who did not receive the therapy. In the United Kingdom, Britain's CFS/ME Working Group felt that cognitive behavioral therapy was one of the key aspects to help improve quality of life and day-to-day functioning for patients. Their research found that among those who could attend therapy, three of four studies found positive overall effect, and improved function and fatigue.

Not everyone is sold on cognitive behavior therapy, however. In the U.K., a patient survey found that only 7 percent of respondents found therapy helpful, 26 percent believed it made them worse, and 67 percent reported "no change."

It's not enough to say that you'll need a more positive attitude to cope better with CFS or fibromyalgia. Sometimes you simply can't will yourself into a better mood or more positive outlook. Looking on the positive side may be partially an innate personality trait but it's also partially a learned behavior, one that cognitive therapy can teach.

In cognitive therapy, you learn how to listen to your automatic thoughts and responses to situations and people, identify those that are unduly negative or distorted, and implement particular techniques to help rebalance your thinking.

Typically, in cognitive therapy, you first identify the event, what is happening objectively. Then you look at how you feel, and rank the emotion in terms of negativity on a scale of 1 to 100, 100 being totally negative.

Then you consider the automatic thoughts you've had in response to the event. The typical negative thoughts fall into several categories and themes:

- **Depression/hopelessness.** The typical response is "Nothing good ever happens to me."
- **Anxiety/fear.** The typical response is "This isn't going to work out."
- **Anger/resentment.** The typical response is "This isn't fair."

After looking at the situation, your emotions, and your automatic thoughts, you then consider your thoughts as hypotheses to be tested, looking for evidence to support or contradict the belief.

■ Lifestyle/Stress

The inability to manage stress can make us more susceptible to illness, and may play a key role in the development of CFS and fibromyalgia. When we're under stress, a variety of physical processes take place. The body's first response is to produce epinephrine and norepinephrine, the "adrenaline rush" hormones that produce the "fight or flight" response. When adrenaline is flooding into the body, the heart races, blood is redirected away from organs and toward muscles, the liver releases sugar, and the abdomen releases fat cells, all designed to provide quick energy. Once the perceived "emergency" is over, the body's systems typically return to normal.

This response is useful if your house is on fire, but it's not appropriate when it's triggered by daily stressors, such as being cut off in traffic, meeting deadlines at work, or worrying about daily challenges. Yet some people with chronic disease and pain go through the day in a constant state of heightened stress.

Some researchers have speculated that dysfunctions in the HPA axis that trigger CFS and fibromyalgia are activated by stress. The adrenal system is meant to step in and provide energy during short periods of high stress, but it's not meant to sustain you for long periods of time. Ultimately, the body is cheated. Elevated cortisol lowers white blood cell levels, reduces immunity, and ultimately, the adrenals end up underfunctioning and producing less cortisol, reducing immunity even further.

Stress also has a variety of negative effects on the body:

• The redirection of blood away from the digestive system inhibits peristalsis, the squeezing motion that moves food along the gastrointestinal tract. This can cause poor absorption of needed nutrients.

• High cortisol can lead to leaky gut syndrome, which allows antigens into the bloodstream and increases the risk of food sensitivities, allergies, and immune dysfunction.

• Stress causes blood sugar imbalances, and the resulting insulin imbalance not only increases the risk of type II diabetes, but it also can cause weight gain.

• Some experts believe that stress may trigger latent viruses at levels high enough to cause low-grade infections but not high enough to be detected using common laboratory tests. The low-grade infections would be sufficient to activate the immune system, decrease immune response and strength, and trigger symptoms.

• Stress may even trigger damage to the body's DNA, which would explain how chronic stress could contribute to CFS, fibromyalgia, and even, over the long term, cancer.

In a study of medical students, for example, researchers found that during exam time, nervous test-takers had an increase in the DNA repair systems that fix cellular damage. This suggests that during the period of stress there was an increase in damaged DNA, and damaged DNA is one factor implicated in cancer.

One recent study dispelled any doubt that mental stress can translate to high levels of harmful hormones. The study of patients with rheumatoid arthritis found that the levels of stress hormones were significantly elevated when patients were under mental stress. But under general anesthesia, the levels dropped substantially. This study illustrated that excessive mental stress had a very specific impact on stress hormone levels, which can then affect the course and control of a disease.

New research has just shown that stress that is imposed on you passively—such as watching violence on television—may weaken your immune system.

One New Jersey study looked at the physical, behavioral, and psychological factors that contribute to the development of CFS. What researchers found after looking at 20 patients and 20 controls, matched for age, sex, and race, was that the level of stress and number of stressful events during the five years immediately before a patient became ill was directly correlated to onset of CFS.

German researchers have found that the hormone ACTH does not work properly in people with CFS. In various stress tests—including preparing for a job interview, pedaling on a stationary bicycle, and injecting of insulin—people diagnosed with CFS had lower levels of ACTH both before and after each test.

■ Stress Management Drugs and Supplements

Debilitating stress may call for the use of prescription antianxiety drugs in some people. Some of the most effective for CFS and fibromyalgia patients include the benzodiazepine class of drugs, including clonazepam (Klonopin), lorazepam (Ativan) and alprazolam (Xanax).

Some patients have reported improvements on low-dose hydrocortisone therapy, but results have been controversial. However, when there is some form of chronic adrenal insufficiency or adrenal fatigue that is contributing to the CFS or fibromyalgia, physiologic doses of replacement cortisol can be therapeutic in some people.

Some herbal supplements may be of help in dealing with mild stress and anxiety, including kava, smaller doses of Dr. Teitelbaum's Revitalizing Sleep Formula, and chamomile tea, among others.

■ Stress Management in Your Life

Whatever is triggering stress, there are also some lifestyle changes that you may need to implement as part of your overall approach to wellness. Here are just a few options to consider:

- Try to eat breakfast and lunch daily.
- Plan to meditate or listen to a relaxation tape for a few minutes each day.
- Instead of drinking coffee all day, switch to herbal tea or water.
- Stop multitasking and instead concentrate on doing one thing at a time.
- Try to get some form of regular exercise.
- Avoid people who are "stress carriers" or "energy vampires."
- Take a "news" fast and avoiding watching news for a day or a week.
- Don't watch the 11 p.m. news.
- Learn how to assertively turn down requests for your time.
- Learn how to breathe properly when you are feeling stressed.
- Adopt a pet.
- Drive less aggressively.
- Resist the temptation to judge or criticize others.
- Be flexible and recognize that things don't always go as you plan.
- Pray, speak to God, your higher power, nature, or your inner guide.

In today's stressful world, be particularly careful about personalizing national and international events. While we have gone through a nonstop media anxiety feeding frenzy with the September 11 tragedy, the war in Afghanistan, the war in Iraq, terror alerts at home, anthrax, snipers, SARS, and more, the reality is that we're constantly barraged with information on threats to our safety. This type of information drives up fear and anxiety, and can shift the body into "fear response." This raises cortisol levels, may increase heart rate and blood pressure, and can lower immune system defenses. Turn off the television. And if you need to know what's going on, get your news from print sources, which are less emotionally charged, rather than from television and radio, where the anxiety of the anchors, reporters, and interview subjects may subtly affect your own level of anxiety.

Of particular importance is to find some way to achieve what's known as the "relaxation response." Harvard physician Herbert Benson, M.D., the nation's foremost mind–body expert, feels that the objective of mind–body medicine is the "relaxation response," his term for the point at which body functions become balanced and actual physiological changes can be observed. In an interview with public radio host Diane Rehm, Dr. Benson articulated his discoveries:

> We have found that when people regularly go into a quiet state, a large percentage of them feel the presence of a power, a force, an energy, God if you will, and they feel that presence is close to them, within them, then these people have fewer medical symptoms. Now, whether or not this is a physiological reaction independent of an external belief system, or whether or not there is indeed something out there, we cannot answer, but from the patient's point of view, they feel better. . . .

There are many different ways to achieve these objectives, from guided imagery to meditation to writing therapy to yoga. Tai chi, breathing, prayer, needlework, and many other techniques also generate this response in different individuals.

Meditation/Mindfulness

One area that is particularly effective at achieving the relaxation response, and actually changing certain aspects of brain function, is meditation.

According to the Center for Integrative Medicine at Thomas Jefferson University Hospital in Philadelphia, meditation training can help patients with chronic illnesses reduce their symptoms and improve their quality of life. Meditation training has also helped patients cope with stress, achieve an improved sense of well-being, reduce body tension, and increase clearness of thinking—all effects that benefit the immune system and help address CFS and fibromyalgia symptoms. Researchers have also established by using magnetic resonance imaging (MRI) that meditation actually activates certain structures in the brain that control the autonomic nervous system.

Another supporter for meditation is the Dalai Lama, who in early 2003 visited the neuroscience laboratory of Dr. Richard Davidson at the University of Wisconsin. Says the Dalai Lama:

> *Using imaging devices that show what occurs in the brain during meditation, Dr. Davidson has been able to study the effects of Buddhist practices for cultivating compassion, equanimity or mindfulness. For centuries Buddhists have believed that pursuing such practices seems to make people calmer, happier and more loving. At the same time they are less and less prone to destructive emotions. According to Dr. Davidson, there is now science to underscore this belief. Dr. Davidson tells me that the emergence of positive emotions may be due to this: Mindfulness meditation strengthens the neurological circuits that calm a part of the brain that acts as a trigger for fear and anger. . . .*

Dr. Davidson has also had success teaching non-Buddhists in high-stress jobs some basic mindfulness techniques over an eight-week period. Dr. Davidson was able to measure that the parts of their brains that help form positive emotions became increasingly active.

Guided Imagery

Guided imagery can be an effective technique for healing. You can use your own imagery, or follow a book, audiotape, or practitioner. If you are feeling stress, you might envision progressively relaxing each part of your body as you lie on a warm sunny beach, or you might envision the body's healing capabilities focusing on a damaged organ.

To try a simple guided-imagery exercise, close your eyes, take several deep full abdominal breaths, and then focus on the symptom that is bothering you. Allow an image—whatever image—to appear that represents your symptom. Don't judge the vision that appears, just accept it and observe it. What feelings do you have about it? Tell the image how you feel about it, silently or out loud. Then visualize that it is answering you, telling you why it's there, what it wants, what it's trying to tell you, or do. Ask the image if it is willing to have your symptom abate. Then decide if you're willing to give it what it wants. Continue the exchange until you feel that you've come to some sort of agreement with the vision.

One particularly effective way to do guided imagery is with audiotapes. I highly recommend the tapes of Belleruth Naparstek, who is considered the leader in guided-imagery work. Belleruth has developed a wonderful "Fibromyalgia & Chronic Fatigue" guided imagery audiotape and CD that is designed to "promote relaxation and the ability to sleep soundly; reduce pain, depression and fatigue; reinforce self-worth and self-care; support balanced functioning of the immune system; help regulate digestive discomfort; heighten motivation and engender faith in the future."

Self-Hypnosis

Another effective technique to generate the relaxation response is self-hypnosis. Research reported in the *Journal of Consulting and Clinical Psychology* found that students who received "hypnotic-relaxation training" did not have a reduction in key immune system components compared to those who did not practice the relaxation techniques. Interestingly, the more often students practiced the relaxation techniques, the stronger their immune response.

Journaling

Have you ever written an e-mail, bulletin board post, diary entry, or letter about something bothering you, and after you were finished felt better about the whole situation? You weren't imagining it—the act of writing about stressful events and situations can actually have a positive impact on your health. In a 1999 study published in the *Journal of the American Medical Association*, researchers reported that some patients with chronic diseases had improvements in their health after writing about major life stresses such as car accidents or the death of a close friend or relative.

The study looked at 112 patients. Each patient spent an hour each day writing, and four months after the study began, almost half of those who wrote about their stresses had experienced significant improvement in their health. The benefit of "downloading" your concerns and stresses, whether by writing a journal or sharing your personal experiences with others who can relate via an online support group, is natural stress reduction. What scientists call "expressive writing" not only gives your mind a place to unload stressful concerns or worries, it can also be a relaxing, or peaceful activity that helps to reduce stress by calming down your system and allowing you to focus better.

Besides straight journaling, or writing-based support group participation, you can also use another technique called a "worry book," in which you draw a line down the page, and list some of your major concerns and stresses on the left and what steps you are taking to try to resolve the problems or solutions you can consider on the right.

"Official worry time" writing is another writing technique that can be helpful. To practice this technique, allow yourself five to fifteen minutes a day of official worry time. Sit down to your journal and in that time allow yourself to freely write down all your fears, stresses, and concerns—as much as you want. Then, at the end of the time frame, close your book or computer file and tell yourself that if you want to worry about something, you will save it up for the next official "worry time."

14

Finding and Working with the Best Practitioners

A Physician who does not admit to the reality of the disease can not be supposed to cure it.
—WILLIAM CULLEN

Having the right practitioner—or team of practitioners—is critical in the treatment of CFS and fibromyalgia.

It's important to think of your practitioners as part of a bigger process, however. One doctor or expert will probably not be the person to provide diagnosis, treatment, and ongoing care over time. More likely, you'll need different practitioners at different points in the course of your condition as well as for the various types of treatment you may need.

To start, you need to be diagnosed. Sometimes diagnosis will come from an astute family practitioner or G.P. In other cases you may need to see a more holistic or complementary medicine expert who is more readily able to recognize a multisystem condition such as CFS or fibromyalgia. Some people are sent by their family doctor to a specialist such as a rheumatologist, who then diagnoses the condition.

According to one survey of almost 300 fibromyalgia patients, on average, the patients had symptoms for almost ten years, and went to an average of almost eight doctor visits before they were diagnosed. Among those surveyed, 60 percent were diagnosed by a rheumatologist, 19 percent by an internist, 12 percent by a family practitioner. The rest were diagnosed by pain specialists, orthopedists, and neurologists.

But after diagnosis, you'll need treatment. At this point, you may be referred to a rheumatologist or pain management specialist.

Or you may go a holistic route. People with CFS/fibromyalgia may want to have at least one reputable holistic/alternative practitioner as part of the health-care team. The multidisciplinary nature of the conditions, the diversity of symptoms, and the need to approach treatment from various angles means that holistic practitioners, with their focus on integrative medicine, may be more suited toward rapid diagnosis and effective treatment of CFS and fibromyalgia.

Here's a review of some of the types of conventional and alternative practitioners whom you may seek out to be part of your health-care team and their areas of specialization.

■ Possible Practitioners on Your Team

General Practitioners/Family Doctors

General practice or family practice doctors typically provide comprehensive health care, and are the physicians of first contact in many situations for patients. The family physician evaluates the patient's total health needs, and provides personal care within one or more fields of medicine. These doctors are prepared to diagnose and treat many conditions, and since the patient–physician relationship is particularly important with G.P.'s and family practitioners, they are familiar with your background and symptoms over time.

Your G.P. or family practice doctor will typically refer you to specialists after ruling out more common reasons for the symptoms.

Some G.P.'s or family practice doctors are holistic and complementary in focus, and concentrate on the whole person and how he or she interacts with the environment rather than on illness, disease, or specific body parts. These doctors, some M.D.'s and some osteopathic physicians (D.O.'s), believe in the prevention of disease when possible, and in dealing with the underlying cause of a problem rather than just treating symptoms. They also focus on integrating complementary modalities—such as herbs, supplements, diet and nutrition, energy work, among others—into their treatment approaches.

Osteopathic Physicians/D.O.'s

Currently, it's estimated that there are more than 30,000 American-educated and -licensed osteopathic physicians practicing in the United States. The majority of osteopathic physicians are in primary care, family medicine, pediatrics, internal medicine, and obstetrics/gynecology. Doctors of osteopathic medicine (D.O.'s) are "complete" physicians, fully trained and licensed to prescribe medication and to perform surgery. Licensed in the same way as other doctors, osteopaths attend an osteopathic medical school, and do internships and residencies.

The main difference is in the philosophy of osteopathy versus that of conventional medicine. Osteopaths typically address people holistically, and instead of treating each symptom separately, look for the overall cause and attempt to treat the whole person. Some osteopaths focus their treatment primarily on osteopathic manipulation, working with the musculoskeletal system as a way to treat illness. There is clear research supporting the use of osteopathic manipulation and techniques for musculoskeletal and nonmusculoskeletal problems. Osteopathic manipulation is particularly useful in terms of muscular and joint pain relief, and some osteopaths specialize in working with fibromyalgia and CFS patients who are experiencing chronic pain.

Internists

Many people don't know what an internist is, but it's a nonsurgical medical specialty that focuses on diseases of internal organs in adults. Internists are typically skilled in managing complex disorders. Some 35 percent are not specialized, and typically act as primary care physicians. Some internists specialize; the subspecialties of internal medicine: cardiology, endocrinology, gastroenterology, hematology, infectious diseases, nephrology, oncology, pulmonary disease, rheumatology, and geriatrics.

Rheumatologists

These doctors specialize in diagnosing and treating arthritis and other diseases of the joints, muscles, and bones, including rheumatoid arthritis, chronic fatigue syndrome, fibromyalgia, osteoarthritis, lupus, and some autoimmune diseases. Rheumatologists have to be detectives, since some of these diseases are difficult to diagnose, and early diagnosis and treatment are important. There is a small subspecialty of holistically oriented rheumatologists who are integrating alternative therapies into Western medical practice.

Neurologists

Neurologists specialize in disorders of the nervous system, including the brain, spinal cord, nerves, and muscles. For some CFS and fibromyalgia patients, a consultation with a neurologist can be a useful part of treatment. The neurologist may be particularly useful when the diagnosis is still being made, since a neurologist has particular expertise in ruling out conditions that may have symptoms similar to CFS and fibromyalgia, including multiple sclerosis, polymyalgia rheumatica (which involves pain in shoulders and hips), polymyositis (which causes arm and leg pain), herniated disks, sciatica, and other neurological conditions.

Infectious Diseases Specialist

An infectious diseases specialist manages the diagnosis and treatment of illnesses caused by microorganisms or germs, including bacteria, viruses, fungi, and parasites. Because their training and experience tends to involve a broad cross section of medicine, these doctors have a more multidisciplinary, investigative focus. Some of these specialists have focused on CFS as their area of expertise.

Pain Management Specialist

A pain management specialist is a doctor who has special training in the management of chronic pain. These doctors typically treat chronic headaches, persistent back pain, cancer pain, arthritis pain, and nerve damage pain, such as diabetic neuropathy, as well as the chronic pain of fibromyalgia and CFS. Pain management specialists have particular expertise in use of various techniques for helping to minimize or treat chronic pain. In particular, they prescribe stronger prescription drugs for pain relief, including opiates, and employ electrical stimulation techniques, behavioral medicine, stress reduction, hypnotherapy, and other approaches.

Endocrinologists

Endocrinologists focus on diseases of the endocrine system and metabolism, including thyroid conditions, hypoglycemia, adrenal problems, and diabetes. A small number specialize in hypothalamic, pituitary and adrenal problems, and in integrative thyroid disease, fibromyalgia, and CFS treatment. Endocrinologists typically have the initials F.A.C.E. after their names, standing for "Fellow, American College of Endocrinology."

Gastroenterologists

These doctors focus on diseases of the esophagus, stomach, liver, pancreas, small intestine, and colon, including irritable bowel syndrome, GERD, and other digestive conditions.

Cardiologists

These doctors are experts in the heart and its actions and diseases. Some cardiologists have specific expertise in the dysautonomia syndromes that affect CFS and fibromyalgia patients, such as neurally mediated hypotension, and are trained in the administration and interpretation of tilt-table testing.

Immunologists

Immunologists study the causes of immunity and immune responses. While many immunologists focus on research, not on patient practice, there are some clinical practitioners who have focused on identifying and treating the immune dysfunctions related to diagnosis and treatment of CFS, and to a lesser extent, fibromyalgia.

Orthopedists

These doctors work on the correction or prevention of skeletal deformities, and some are involved in conditions such as rheumatoid arthritis and other conditions that affect the joints. There are some orthopedists who specialize in treating fibromyalgia.

Traditional Chinese Medicine Practitioners

Traditional Chinese medicine (TCM) originated some 4,000 years ago, and its principles are based on health in terms of the individual and his or her surroundings. Central to that balance is *qi* (pronounced "chee"), which is translated as "vital energy" or "life force." Qi flows through the body via pathways known as meridians, and is exchanged with the body's surroundings. A body is in optimal health when there is free and balanced flow of qi. In addition to qi, TCM relies on the concept of yin and yang, the interdependent opposites, representing different organs and health aspects.

TCM diagnostic techniques include observation, listening, questioning, and palpation, including feeling special pulse qualities and sensitivity of body parts. TCM treatments include diet, exercises such as tai chi and the qi gong breathing, herbal preparations, acupuncture, acupressure massage, physical therapy, and moxibustion (use of heat at specific energy points on the body). In the U.S., acupuncture has become an increasingly established practice, both as part of TCM and even more so on its own. Americans make more than ten million trips a year to acupuncturists, and more than three thousand conventionally trained U.S. physicians also practice acupuncture. TCM and acupuncture have been proven effective in some chronic pain and energy problems.

When choosing an acupuncturist, be sure to see someone who is licensed and certified, whether a doctor or not. For physicians, top certification is from the American Academy of Medical Acupuncture (AAMA). Acupuncturists who are not doctors can receive credentials known as a Diplomate in Acupuncture (Dipl.Ac.). They may be called Licensed Acupuncturist (L.Ac. or Lic.Ac.), Registered Acupuncturist (R.Ac.), Certified Acupuncturist (C.A.), Acupuncturist, Doctor of Oriental Medicine (D.O.M.) or Doctor of Acupuncture (D.Ac.). Each state has its own specific requirements for practice of acupuncture. Either see a licensed acupuncturist or one who is nationally certified from an organization such as the National Certification Commission for Acupuncture and Oriental Medicine (NCCAOM).

Naturopaths/Herbalists

When it comes to finding the right herbal practitioner, it's particularly important that you find someone who has long-standing experience, a good reputation, and who has demonstrated clear knowledge of CFS and fibromyalgia. The last thing you want to do is end up with a multilevel vitamin salesperson claiming to be an herbal medicine practitioner! Your best chance for success in finding an experienced herbalist or naturopathic practitioner is to seek out a member of the American Herbalists Guild or a recommended licensed naturopathic physician.

Ayurvedic Practitioners

Ayurveda (pronounced "Ah-yuhr-VAY-duh") has been the traditional medicine of India for more than five thousand years, and is probably the oldest medical system in existence. *Ayurveda* is a Sanskrit word that means "science of life" or "life knowledge," and is based on the premise that the body naturally seeks harmony and balance. In ayurveda, disease represents emotional imbalance, unhealthy lifestyle, toxins in the body, and most especially, imbalances. Proper balancing is accomplished through food and diet, herbs, meditation and breathing, massage, and even yoga poses to ensure that energy is flowing.

Some naturopaths and homeopaths offer aspects of ayurvedic treatment or incorporate ayurvedic herbal preparations as part of their treatments. There are also purely ayurvedic practitioners. There is no official "licensing" to be an ayurvedic practitioner, so you should ask where and how long a practitioner was trained, how long he or she has been practicing ayurveda, and how much of his or her practice is purely ayurveda.

Chiropractors

Chiropractors—doctors of chiropractic—focus on the structural, spinal, musculoskeletal, neurological, vascular, nutritional, emotional, and environmental aspects of health. Chiropractic treatment, being drugfree and nonsurgical science, typically involves adjustment, alignment, and manipulation of the joints and tissues, particularly, the spinal column. One late 1990s study by the Gallup Organization determined that 90 percent of chiropractic patients rated their treatment as effective, and 80 percent were satisfied with the treatment they received and felt that most of their expectations were met.

Physical Therapists

A physical therapist is someone who treats injury, pain, or dysfunction with exercises, massage, and other physical treatments. They are sometimes called physiotherapists. Physical therapists design programs that may include muscle strengthening, flexibility and conditioning, and pain management. Treatment may include a specific exercise or rehabilitation program and various modalities such as heat, ultrasound, electrical stimulation, ice, a home exercise program, range-of-motion exercises, or other treatments.

Manual Healers/Bodyworkers

Manual healing and bodywork encompass so many different forms that it's hard to even list them all. A few include Swedish massage, trigger point massage (myotherapy, neuromuscular massage therapy), Rolfing, Trager, Alexander technique, and Feldenkrais. Practitioners of reflexology and acupressure stimulate points so as to clear energy pathways that appear to be blocked. And there are many kinds of energetic work, such as Reiki and therapeutic touch, in which the therapist is a conduit for healing energy that is directed to the patient through the therapist's hands, sometimes without actually touching the client. There are different licensing and accreditation requirements for each type of bodywork. Many specialty areas—such as Rolfing and Feldenkrais—offer separate certification. Some states and areas license massage therapists. The main certification to look for, however, is N.C.T.M.B., which is granted by the National Certification Board for Therapeutic Massage & Bodywork, after completion of five hundred hours of training and passage of an exam.

■ Finding a Great New Practitioner

Finding the right practitioners is truly the most essential step in your effort to get the best possible treatment—or even in receiving a correct diagnosis in the first place. To find great practitioners, there are a few key steps to follow.

Qualities and Features

Decide what qualities and features you are looking for in a doctor or practitioner. Most people are willing to spend time finding a good plumber, accountant, or babysitter; you need to make even more of an effort to find the right health-care experts. Before you start the selection process, consider your main priorities and criteria:

Male/female. It's important to consider whether or not a male or female doctor is best for you. Men and women doctors tend to have different ways of interacting with patients. Women doctors, for example, tend to spend more time with patients than their male colleagues. One study found that women spent, on average, eight minutes (or 29 percent) longer with patients than male doctors. In Dutch research, almost 33 percent of visits with female physicians were longer than ten minutes versus about 26 percent with male doctors. Generally, studies suggest that women doctors tend to be more successful at involving patients in decisions and explaining things.

Cost/coverage. For some people, going outside the HMO or insurance plan is simply not a financial option. It's helpful to make this decision up front, so you can narrow your search accordingly. If you are limited to selecting doctors from a preapproved list provided by your HMO or health plan, you may want to start by asking your HMO plan or insurance company if they offer any help in choosing from their lists or if they have more information on available doctors. Otherwise, many of the other resources we'll discuss here can be used to help "qualify" the doctors you do have available via your HMO or insurance plan.

Experience. How many years of experience you want may depend on your preferences. Younger doctors may be more open to things like alternative medicine, whereas older doctors might be more set in their ways but be more seasoned, experienced, and have a better bedside manner.

Credentials. In some cases, you may want a doctor who graduated from a top conventional or osteopathic medical school. This isn't always an indicator of a good doctor, but the top-echelon medical schools usually manage to weed out some of the worst students.

Certification. Being "board certified" means a doctor has had several additional years of training in a particular specialty and passed a competency exam. Again, this doesn't guarantee that the doctor will be a success for you, but you're getting assurance of extra education in the particular specialty.

Some other important factors include

- **Record.** Some people want to make sure there are no disciplinary actions filed against a doctor, and there are ways to evaluate this.
- **Cutting edge.** Some people want a doctor who is innovative and on the cutting edge, who reads all the journals and health reports and keeps up with developments.
- **Conventional or alternative focus.** Some people balk at having a practitioner who suggests acupuncture or herbal remedies, and others, for example, wouldn't want a practitioner who *wasn't* open to alternative therapies.

- **Flexibility.** Some people want a doctor who has evening or weekend hours, or who can see patients on short notice, or who will consult by phone.
- **Success.** Most people want a doctor who has successfully treated other patients with CFS and/or fibromyalgia. This may be information you can get only from other patients, or perhaps from another doctor.
- **Recommendations.** You might want to talk to other patients who are satisfied customers of this practitioner. If a practitioner is not willing to provide patient references, look somewhere else.
- **Referrals or peer recommendations.** You might want a doctor who has been recommended by other doctors. There are a variety of sources of this information that you can access.

Identify Candidates

Identify several candidates. Once you know what type of doctor or practitioner you are looking for, ask friends and relatives, medical specialists, and other health professionals for the names of practitioners they highly recommend. Ask about the person's experiences, and what they like or don't like about a practitioner.

Once you've narrowed down your selections and have a short list of possible practitioners, it's time to have a brief screening interview by phone, during which you might want to ask the following sorts of questions:

- Are you accepting new patients and, if so, is a referral required?
- Are you an individual or group practice? If I have an appointment with you, is there a possibility I may be seen by another doctor without advance notice?
- Who covers for you when you're unavailable?
- On average, how long does a patient have to wait for an appointment? (How long in advance must I make an appointment?)

- Do you charge for missed appointments?
- Do you accept patient phone calls? Do you restrict them to any particular time of day? How soon do you typically return calls? Do you have your nurses return calls on your behalf? Do you charge for phone calls?
- Is advice given over the phone?
- Do you accept patient e-mails?
- Do you accept patient faxes?
- What are your customary fees?
- Do you accept my health insurance coverage or Medicare?
- Is full payment (or deductibles, co-payments) required at the time of the appointment?
- Do you take the time to explain treatment options, answer questions, and generally involve patients in their own treatment?
- Are lab work and X rays performed in the office? Do you send your blood out for tests or do you perform them in-house?
- What hours are you available?
- Do you have experience helping to successfully support disability claims for CFS/fibromyalgia?
- Do you refer patients to alternative treatments?
- Can you provide several patient references I can check out?

If a practitioner's office isn't interested in at least providing you with some of this information in advance, I'd suggest moving on. Practitioners who don't recognize that patients are clients to whom they provide a service often aren't productive in the long run.

Verify Credentials

Look at reference sources for verification. The Official American Board of Medical Specialties Directory of Board Certified Medical Specialists is available at many libraries, and they have a free online search service as well. See Resources at the back of the book for more information.

Don't assume, however, that just because a doctor is on a hospital or magazine's Best Doctors list or a practitioner is well known in your area that the person is right for you.

Learn About the Doctors

Learn more about the doctors you are considering. Call their offices. The office staff can be a good source of information about the doctor's education and qualifications, office policies, and payment procedures. Pay attention to the office staff—you may have to deal with them often! You may want to set up an appointment to talk with a doctor. He or she is likely to charge you for such a visit.

There are other questions about your potential practitioner that unfortunately can't usually be answered until you are a patient. You may be able to get some ideas from other patients, but it's more likely you'll need to assess the doctor firsthand. However, keep your ears and eyes open when talking to other patients, when talking on the phone to the office, or during the initial visit, since some of the answers to these questions can be answered fairly early on:

- Does your doctor/practitioner patiently explain reasons for all tests and treatments?
- Does your doctor/practitioner offer you options?
- Does your doctor/practitioner seem interested in educating you, or just in giving orders to be followed?
- Does your doctor/practitioner encourage you to participate in decisions about your health care?
- Does your doctor/practitioner believe in alternative or complementary therapies?
- Does your doctor/practitioner take time to learn about you, your background, your lifestyle, and how you truly feel?
- Does your doctor/practitioner really listen?
- Does your doctor/practitioner answer your questions satisfactorily?

• Do your doctor/practitioner's receptionists, nurses, and other staff treat you and other patients politely and respectfully?

• Does your doctor/practitioner and his/her staff let you dress and undress in private?

• Does your doctor/practitioner or his/her staff gossip or share private information about other patients?

• Does your doctor/practitioner admit or indicate that he/she just "isn't comfortable" with assertive or informed patients?

• Does your doctor/practitioner take an authoritarian or dictatorial approach to the doctor–patient relationship?

• Does your doctor/practitioner become irritated, act impatient, or ignore you when you ask for further explanation of your diagnosis, procedures to be performed, or drugs being prescribed?

• Does your doctor/practitioner return phone calls within a reasonable amount of time, or tell you that he/she has left messages or tried to call when it's evident he/she hasn't?

• Does your doctor/practitioner keep you waiting and usually run late for your appointments?

• When you mention some major health finding you heard about on the evening news, does your doctor/practitioner seem at all aware of it?

• Will your doctor/practitioner read anything you provide him/her as far as background information?

• Does your doctor/practitioner categorically dismiss the Internet as a source of quack information?

Make Your Selection and Evaluate

The final step is to make your selection. After your first appointment, evaluate whether you feel comfortable and can work well with this doctor. If you weren't satisfied, consider visiting one of the other doctors on your short list.

■ Effective Communication with Your Practitioners

With a chronic disease, it is particularly important to maintain open, effective communication with your practitioners. There are a variety of ways you can help optimize this communication.

Keep Good Medical Records

You should keep as complete a medical record as possible. Your information can be maintained in a notebook, a binder, on the computer, or in folders. The main concern is keeping track of appointments, copies of test results, and other pertinent information, including

- **Doctor/practitioner information.** Include the name, address, phone, fax, and e-mail addresses for every doctor and practitioner you see—even those you only see periodically. Keep track of receptionists' names. And also store directions to offices you don't visit frequently.
- **Pharmacy information.** Include the prescription numbers and number of refills available for all current prescriptions, plus phone numbers for your pharmacy or pharmacies.
- **Lab/treatment facility information.** Include the name, address, and phone number of any labs or treatment facilities (radiology labs, testing locations, physical therapists, etc.).

Your records/health diary should also keep track of your key health events, including illnesses, surgeries, and other pertinent information. A detailed health diary would include

- Dates of visits to the doctor
- Dates when you've received any injections, vaccinations, or special treatments
- Dates and locations of diagnostic procedures

- Dates starting and stopping a medication, and dosage levels
- Blood test results—ask for a photocopy for your folder
- Major emotional and physical stresses

You can also keep copies of your Pain and Fatigue Daily Diary/Checklist (from chapter 5) and include them in your records.

One of the most important things you need to do is to request, review, and keep copies of your tests. One way to facilitate this is to give your practitioners self-addressed stamped envelopes in which to send test results—they appreciate it and it makes the point you are serious. Ask for copies of the original test results, not the doctor's handwritten summaries of the information. Include blood work, X-ray reports, pathology and special study results, typed consultation reports from specialists, all heart testing and procedures, discharge summary and operative summary if hospitalized.

Preparing for Your Appointment

A productive doctor's appointment is one during which you have a chance to cover your key concerns with the practitioner. In many offices, time is at a premium, so a successful appointment requires advance preparation. Some tips:

- Write down the names and dosages of all medications—including supplements and herbs—that you are taking.
- Prioritize your concerns. Studies have shown that patients will go to the doctor with several complaints, but will often wait to mention the one that is of most concern until the end of the visit, when the doctor is about to leave the exam room. If your doctor knows all the specific concerns you have when he or she enters, then you can have an appropriate discussion.
- Ideally, once you've considered your main concerns, write them down, and bring a written list of problems, with the most important problem listed first. Put your concerns into the form of

an agenda for your visit, and bring two copies, one for the practitioner. Be sure you include on your agenda all key questions, concerns, or unusual health symptoms.

• Share your research ahead of time. If you have articles or information—more than your one-page list of concerns—that you would like to share with your doctor, mail or fax it ahead of time, with a note regarding the date and time of your appointment and the fact that you'd like to discuss this at that time. If you bring these materials to the appointment without sending them in advance, your doctor may not have time to review them, or may spend the entire appointment reading rather than communicating with you.

• Get in business mode. Act as if your appointment is a business meeting. You're the client; the doctor is the "contractor," so to speak. Doctors treat patients more respectfully when the patients dress professionally for the appointment, and when patients stay calm, relaxed, and unemotional, and do not act apologetic or passive.

• Be sure to arrive on time. If you arrive in advance, don't spend time reading old magazines, spend the time reviewing your agenda and mentally preparing for your appointment.

• Take notes. It's hard to remember what the doctor says after an appointment, so jot down notes, names of things, instructions and other information, so you have a reference. Tape-record your conversation with the practitioner's permission if you aren't confident that you will remember everything the doctor says.

• Bring a friend. This can help you feel more relaxed with the doctor. If you doctor gives you a hard time about having a friend with you, this is a red flag. You're the patient, you're paying the bill, and you should be able to decide whom you'd like in the examining room with you. Choose a friend who is able to speak up but is diplomatic. Friends who are health professionals—or even doctors themselves—can be of particular help. Be sure your friend knows the agenda for the appointment, so he or she can remind you of points to cover and can help you remember details of what your doctor said or agreed to do.

• Ask questions. It's important to ask questions at your appointment when you don't understand something or want to further explore solutions. This advice is particularly important for men. Studies have shown that men tend to internalize health fears and concerns, and even when worried, are reluctant to admit to concerns or problems. One study found that the average man asked his doctor no questions during an office visit versus the average woman, who asked six.

More than anything, remember that your doctor needs to be your partner in wellness decisions, so ideally, you need to find a compassionate, informed practitioner who is willing to work with you—not dictate to you—to find the right diagnosis, treatment, and solutions that will allow you to achieve optimal health.

■ Problem Solving with Challenging Doctors

Sometimes you may not have the option to change doctors. When you are truly stuck, and geographic, financial, or HMO factors have limited you to a particular practitioner, you may need more assertive tactics to get the diagnosis and treatment you deserve.

Document

Be sure to bring your CFS/Fibromyalgia Risks and Symptoms Checklist (see chapter 4) to your first appointment, and ask that it be included in your medical chart. If your doctor refuses to refer you to a specialist or conduct key tests, provide another copy of the checklist and put a note on it indicating that the doctor has refused referral/testing, etc. Ask the doctor to sign and date it, and have a copy put in your file and a copy given to you. Send a copy to your HMO or insurance company's ombudsman or consumer liaison, along with your request that referral or testing be approved.

Write Letters

Write a simple letter that states that for the various reasons listed (and list them), you have specifically requested referral or particular testing and that this doctor has refused. Ask the doctor to sign it and place a copy in your chart. Keep a signed copy in your own file as well. (You can then use this copy with the HMO in your request for a referral to another doctor, if needed.) Most doctors will give you the referral or order tests rather than officially document their decision to refuse a patient's request.

Complain

While it's a last resort, it is sometimes appropriate to complain. According to one survey, dissatisfied patients who threatened their doctor with negative publicity or said they might file a complaint could demonstrably affect their course of treatment. According to the research, 44 percent of physicians will act in a defensive way to protect themselves legally when dealing with a case where relatives threaten to go to the press if the doctor doesn't order further tests for a family member's chest pain. Without the threat, only 30 percent would order the tests. In the same study, 57 percent of doctors would make a referral for a patient with severe headaches who threatened to file a formal medical complaint if not referred to a neurologist versus only 25 percent of doctors who were not threatened. So it may be a more hard-charging tactic, but if you have no recourse in terms of getting a new primary care practitioner, consider filing a formal complaint to get the diagnosis or treatment you need.

■ When It's Time to Make a Change: Signs That You Need a New Doctor

When you're dealing with a chronic disease, it's very likely that at some point you will need a new doctor. Making the decision to find a new doctor is actually far more difficult than most of us might think. Your relationship with doctors is an intensely personal one, and it's not easy to sever that connection—let alone find the right match—particularly when limited by specialties available, geography, HMOs, and insurance, among other factors.

You may also feel a bit intimidated by your doctor, and feel that once you have a relationship with a particular practitioner, you shouldn't switch, or you'll offend the doctor if you do.

Remember, in a doctor–patient relationship *you* are the client, and the doctor is providing a service. And if that service is not meeting your needs, the best thing you can do for your health is to find the doctor who *will* meet your needs.

When you have a chronic disease, you may visit your doctor frequently. Your relationship with your doctor is the foundation of your health and well-being. The wrong doctor may take away any or all opportunity for you to return to wellness and optimal health.

How do you know when it's time for a new practitioner? Here are some signs.

Your practitioner doesn't respond to calls or faxes.

Maybe you find yourself leaving message after message, but not getting a return call for days, or at all. Or you may end up going several days without a prescribed medicine because your doctor won't call back to okay your refill request. These are signs that patient care and follow-up are not priorities for this practitioner.

Your practitioner's office staff members are unresponsive, disorganized, or rude.

Maybe when you talk to the practitioner, it's clear that your messages don't reach him or her. Or again, you have to go without needed prescription medications because office staff haven't called in a refill or checked with the doctor despite your requests. Office staff members may act rude or dismissive on the phone or in person. They may talk about other patients in front of you. The office may regularly make billing mistakes, overcharge you, or lose paperwork. Or you may show up for a scheduled appointment only to be told that there's no record of your appointment.

Your practitioner tends to dismiss symptoms as "all in your head."

Unfortunately, when facing conditions as complicated as CFS and fibromyalgia, less prepared practitioners may tend to resort to the erroneous assumption that the conditions are psychosomatic, or that symptoms are "in your head." Too quick a tendency to start indiscriminately handing out antidepressants and ignoring physical symptoms is a sign that you may have a practitioner who doesn't understand CFS or fibromyalgia.

Hannah describes her experiences:

I have encountered many mediocre doctors who don't have the mental firepower to recognize an uncommon illness and don't know what to do about it. They ignore things they don't understand, or assign them a "wastebasket diagnosis"—which means, "It's all in your head." Doctors and other people have told me I look just fine, the tests were negative, there's nothing wrong, just pull yourself up by your bootstraps, forget about it, everything's fine, here just take this supplement, take lots of iron or vitamin C, think positive thoughts, you're afraid of success, etc. I have frequently wished I could let them spend some quality time with me inside my body (on a day of my choosing, of course). They'd be screaming to be let out in a few minutes.

Your practitioner dismisses the Internet, books, and support groups as sources of quackery and nonsense.

According to one professional survey, people seeking information about medical procedures are more than twice as likely to get it from the Internet as they are from their doctors. In this era of HMO-limited office visits and harried doctors, patient-oriented health information has never been more important. Does your doctor refuse to look at any information you bring in from the Internet or ignore any books that you bring in?

Some physicians truly do not have an understanding of what is available on the Internet. They don't realize that everything from their favorite medical journals, to the National Library of Medicine database, to most of the major patient and professional organizations have extensive Web sites and online publications. Or they don't realize that a book's author does not need an M.D. after his or her name in order for the information and advice to be valid and pertinent. If your doctor categorically dismisses things you learn in books, on the Internet, or in support groups as unproven or quackery, and isn't willing to at least discuss them with you rationally, then it's a sign that your doctor is threatened by new information.

Your practitioner is unwilling to explore your ideas.

Some practitioners are not particularly open to ideas when you are the one raising them, or don't have the time or talent to explore your symptoms or concerns further. If you request a particular test, for example, does your doctor say "You don't have that condition" and refuse to order the test? If you asked for a different drug, or a new drug based on something you'd read, would your doctor usually refuse without exploring the possible benefits? Or if you bring up a symptom or concern, is your doctor quick to assume that it's just part of your condition and not worth further exploration or separate workup and treatment?

Your practitioner is in it solely for the profits.

If you have one of those practitioners whose office is filled with bottles and jars of expensive vitamins, supplements, powders, potions, books, videos, or other materials for sale, and you get a hard pitch from the practitioner or his/her staff to buy, buy, buy, that's not a good sign. Maybe your practitioner regularly recommends certain products that you can *only* get from him/her. Or the doctor may be pushing you to sign up for multiple sessions per week of his or her particular pet treatment—anything from chelation, to specialized physical therapy, to hyperbaric therapy that is provided at his/her office. It's one thing to have some products and services on hand for your convenience, but claims that the brand of supplement *they* sell, or heavily marked up vitamins and supplements that you could buy for far less at a local vitamin or health food store are all warning signs. Another key warning sign is if you periodically or even frequently find surprises in your bill—charges that you don't understand and that you can't get reasonably explained by the practitioner and staff.

Your practitioner doesn't listen.

Unfortunately, some practitioners make it pretty clear that they are not paying attention. The practitioner may pop in and out of the examining room or office to take phone calls while you are having an appointment. Or your doctor may sit at his or her desk and read, go through mail, or type on the computer while you are having an appointment. One warning sign is that your practitioner is asking you the same questions over and over, indicating that he or she doesn't remember what you've said.

Your practitioner promises more than he or she can deliver.

When it comes to CFS and fibromyalgia, you need to be particularly careful about doctors who promise more than they can deliver. Too much talk of cures or astounding success may rightfully make you skeptical.

Gretchen sums it up well:

My primary complaint of the medical community is that when they don't know what else to do, or how else they can help, I wish they would just say that they don't know. I have more respect for the doctors I have had that have told me they don't know what else to test for, or how else to treat me, than those doctors who get angry and disrespectful of me. I have had so many doctors tell me that they know that others haven't been able to treat me, but they have the answer, they have the cure, and why am I not more excited. But I have learned. It is not that I have lost all hope; hope is what has kept me alive, what keeps me going, but I no longer hope to be completely well right now. I know this makes doctors really angry, but it isn't that I'm discouraged or depressed. After 10 years I have learned that I do have to be realistic to keep my hope alive. Getting my hopes up every time, and being crushed when things didn't work was a large part of my depression. You can't be this sick for this long and not have to fight that battle at some point.

Your practitioner doesn't see the bigger picture.

With chronic conditions, there's a danger that the practitioner doesn't really ever sit down and put together the bigger picture of your health situation. This is the same reason some people have to return as many as seven times before a diagnosis of CFS or fibromyalgia is made. Some warning signs that your practitioner is missing the big picture: He or she acts as if each appointment is totally independent of the last, and doesn't remember symptoms or conditions you've had in the past. The doctor may never pull out your chart and review your history, even for a few moments. Or you may even get the sense that your doctor never has read your chart or history, particularly if you're getting shuttled to different doctors thanks to an HMO.

A pharmaceutical company influences your doctor.

Does your doctor have mousepads, pens, pencils, prescription pads, calendars, mugs, patient information literature, wall charts and posters, and other paraphernalia with drug or pharmaceutical company logos plastered on them? This is a sign that your doctor is regularly visited by the drug company representatives, and may even have a relationship with the drug company. Many doctors receive grants, speaking engagement fees, sponsorships, and many other types of payment that build and solidify the relationships between the doctors and particular drugs the companies want them to prescribe more heavily. A warning sign: when your doctor refuses to allow you to switch to competing brands of drugs, and fails to provide a rational reason other than "This drug is just better."

Your practitioner is arrogant or rude.

Is your doctor one of those men or women who truly think they are "holier than thou" and acts accordingly? Does your practitioner make you wait for extremely long periods of time, but never apologizes for making you wait? Would your doctor *never* say, "I don't know the answer?" These are warning signs that your practitioner is heavy on the arrogance and ego, and short on consideration and compassion. Other warnings: a practitioner that interrupts you or acts impatient when you are speaking, or talks to you in a condescending or patronizing way.

Nancy describes some of her encounters:

Since I've had CFIDS for nearly 20 years, I've had countless encounters with unsympathetic or condescending physicians. The worst are those healthcare providers who tell you that they KNOW what CFIDS is but really don't. I had a bad experience recently with a physical therapist who implied he was going to "fix" my back problem, however, he gave no regard to my CFIDS because in reality he felt it was purely psychological. Needless to say, after one session with him, I relapsed terribly. Fortunately, my CFIDS specialist sent this physical therapist some information to enlighten him on the limitations of exercise, etc. when dealing with a CFIDS patient. However, I never returned for additional treatment.

Ultimately, the above issues are signs that your practitioner is not your partner in wellness, and that is critical for CFS and fibromyalgia patients. Ideally, you want your practitioners to be smart, up-to-date, open-minded, able to quickly diagnose you, and then cure you—fast! Sometimes this happens. But more often than not, it's not the case. The best he or she may be able to do is help minimize your CFS and fibromyalgia symptoms, optimize your health as best as possible, or help you learn coping and management skills. That is why a partner is so essential—someone who will work with you to explore the situation, help you get the best possible diagnosis, explore treatments, fine-tune treatments as necessary, all the time working *in partnership* with you. A practitioner who is your partner will treat you with courtesy and respect, will listen to you, and will incorporate you into the decision-making process.

Remember, of course, that there is no perfect practitioner. A great practitioner or doctor may have almost every quality you want, but be a bit more costly than you'd like. Or you may have found someone you love, but he or she always runs late and keeps you waiting. Or the practitioner is so popular there is a six-month waiting list for routine appointments—and forget about getting squeezed in on short notice. You can't expect perfection! But do expect a practitioner who will make his or her best effort on your behalf. You and your health deserve it!

15

Creating Your Plan

It does not take much strength to do things,
but it requires great strength to decide what to do.

—CHOW CHING

Putting together and implementing a plan to deal with your CFS or fibromyalgia may be one of the biggest challenges you face as part of your condition. As you can see from the previous chapters in this book, there are dozens of options to consider, many drugs and supplements to choose from, and a variety of different types of practitioners who can serve as your partners, guides, and advisers, many with quite different perspectives on what offers the most promise in treating your condition. It is daunting to decide how to proceed.

Keep in mind that putting together your plan is a bit like dividing up a pie, with each slice representing a different technique or approach you can take. In deciding how big each piece will be, you're choosing what amount of time, energy, money, and resources you will devote to that particular technique.

There is no magic formula to tell you ahead of time which mix of approaches, drugs, supplements, and lifestyle changes will work for you. Even the vast majority of practitioners who have worked with thousands of CFS and fibromyalgia patients will tell you that they don't have a surefire "formula" for success. Rather they tend to advocate a "person-centered approach" to treating CFS and fibromyalgia. Because these conditions are the result of complex interactions of many different factors, the treatments are likely also to be fairly complex combinations of many different treatment approaches.

There is, therefore, no single "protocol" that can address the health challenges of everyone with CFS or fibromyalgia. Instead, the person-centered approach takes inventory of symptoms, lifestyle, and the demands of daily life, and chooses from a menu of options the approach that best addresses the person's unique requirements. Then, over time, as results are gauged, the program can be modified and tweaked to meet changing physical needs and emphasize what's most effective.

■ What Works?

In 1999, the Fibromyalgia Network looked at a variety of recommended approaches by different CFS and fibromyalgia practitioners. Just a partial list of practitioners reads like a *Who's Who* of the nation's top experts in CFS and fibromyalgia, including

- Robert Bennett, M.D., a Portland, Oreg., rheumatologist
- Paul Brown, M.D., Ph.D., a Seattle rheumatologist
- Paul Cheney, a North Carolina-based physician and CFS/ fibromyalgia expert
- Daniel Clauw, M.D., a Washington, D.C., rheumatologist
- Steve Fanto, M.D., a Phoenix pain specialist/physiatrist
- Charles Lapp, M.D., a Charlotte, N.C., internal medicine specialist
- Mark Pellegrino, M.D., a Canton, Ohio-based physiatrist

- Richard Podell, M.D., a Springfield, N.J., alternative medicine specialist
- Thomas Romano, M.D., Ph.D., a Wheeling, W.Va., rheumatologist
- Jacob Teitelbaum, M.D., an Annapolis, Md.-based physician and CFS/fibromyalgia expert
- Daniel Wallace, M.D., a Los Angeles-based rheumatologist

While each practitioner has his own particular area of emphasis, they tend to share a multidisciplinary approach to CFS and fibromyalgia. Their focus? Several key objectives include:

- Break the pain cycle
- Ensure uninterrupted, restorative sleep
- Improve mental focus and cognition
- Increase energy, reduce fatigue
- Increase activity levels and function

The approaches they typically recommend include some or all of the following treatments, to varying degrees:

- Gentle, nonimpact exercise when possible
- Pain management, including use of opioids
- A combination of sleep hygiene and sleep supplements/medications to ensure optimal sleep
- Antidepressant therapy for sleep, pain, mood, and cognition
- Injection therapies, such as trigger point injections, Botox, and ketamine for pain
- Acupuncture, for pain relief
- Physical therapy, massage, craniosacral therapy, and myofascial release for pain relief
- Cognitive behavioral therapy when needed
- Relaxation, stress reduction, and management

- General nutritional support and specific nutritional support for deficiencies

In one analysis, almost fifty different studies involving people with fibromyalgia found that nondrug approaches generally were superior to drug treatments in reducing symptoms and improving daily function.

In another survey of nearly 300 patients with fibromyalgia, patients rated various therapies that have been effective. According to patients, effective therapies included pain, sleep, and antidepressant medications, heat therapy, water therapy, physical therapy, massage, exercise, pacing of activities, and avoiding chemicals and allergenic foods.

But again, what works for you will be unique to you, and the best thing you can do is to embark on the process with an open mind and a willingness to adjust your plan as you go.

■ Plan Essentials

There are some things that, no matter what specific approaches you take, should be an essential part of your plan.

Trust Your Instincts

More than anything else, it's essential that you trust your own instincts. You will be relying on your instincts to help guide you toward the practitioners, approaches, and treatments that make the most sense to you. Your decisions may not be made on anything more than a gut feeling, or a sense, after reading or hearing about a particular approach, that "Wow, that just sounds so *right!*" Or you may choose to find a practitioner who inspires your utmost trust, confidence, faith, and hope, and follow his or her direction. Instinct comes into play there as well, because some of the best practitioners are combining their own instincts, applying the "art" of medicine to making decisions about a complex and rarely clear-cut treatment approach.

Trust yourself, trust your instincts, and trust what your body is trying to tell you.

Start with a Positive Attitude

One of the most essential things you can do is to outfit yourself with a positive attitude. In sixteen studies it was shown that patients who have positive expectations about recovery usually do recover well, and are likely to have a better outcome than people who do not have positive expectations.

Beryl finds that a positive attitude is a help to her health:

I work very hard at living one day at a time, not dwelling on negative thoughts, about those days and months of untreated pain when this all began, appreciating each day's beauty and gifts, and try to remember to be thankful just for each day that I have.

Research published in the *Journal of Personality and Social Psychology* in 2001 found that a positive emotional state at an early age could actually help ward off disease and even prolong life. The experts behind the research theorize that the more optimistic a person is, the less stress that person puts on his or her body over time. When there is less stress, the body has more resources to devote to healing.

One interesting study looked at 660 people over fifty evaluated over more than twenty years, gauging their agreement with or disagreement with statements such as "Things keep getting worse as I get older," "I have as much pep as I did last year," and "I am as happy now as I was when I was younger." Researchers found that those who viewed aging as a positive experience lived, on average, 7.5 years longer than those who took a darker view.

Another study linked optimism and longevity. Mayo Clinic psychiatrist Toshihiko Maruta reviewed the results of psychological tests given to more than 800 people in the early 1960s and identified 197 of them as pessimists. Dr. Maruta found that in any given year, the pessimists had a risk of death 19 percent greater than average.

Follow Your Bliss/Find Your Passion

In his book *Three Steps To Happiness!: Healing Through Joy*, CFS/fibromyalgia practitioner Jacob Teitelbaum, M.D., tells everyone, including patients with chronic illness, to "follow your bliss." As Dr. Teitelbaum says,

> . . . [E]motions and feelings are our soul's guidance system . . . keeping our attention on and doing what feels good helps us get to where we truly want to go and be who we truly are.

One CFS patient who has truly followed her bliss is best-selling author Laura Hillenbrand. Her first book, *Seabiscuit*, took four years to write, but went on to become a number one bestseller, and was made into a documentary and a major feature film.

For years, Hillenbrand persevered, conducting almost all her research from bed, by phone and online. Her symptoms were so bad that there were weeks on end when she did all her writing while flat on her back with eyes closed, bedridden due to debilitating fatigue and vertigo.

Hillenbrand told me in an interview that she always knew she would be a writer—she had a great passion for it from a young age. At the same time, after writing an article about Seabiscuit, she also developed a passion to tell Seabiscuit's whole story. Those twin passions drove her to persevere through the incredibly difficult and taxing writing process. As exhausting as it was, writing was a tremendous release from the day-to-day reality of her disabling CFS. "I escaped my body," says Hillenbrand. "It was exhilarating because I loved the story."

Seabiscuit's run became metaphorical for her own effort to write this book. In various interviews with her college alumni magazine and CNN, Hillenbrand said:

> *Writing is my greatest escape. The only time I approach being unaware of physical suffering is when I am absorbed in my writing. I have chosen to write about these people and this horse in part because of the vigor of their lives. . . . I am the ultimate stationary person and these are the ultimate in vigorous people. It's been very therapeutic.*

Hillenbrand has tried a number of different treatments, but has not found any approach that has offered her any substantial relief. For now, while she frequently speaks out on behalf of CFS awareness and her fellow patients, she prefers to shift her personal focus away from her illness. Hillenbrand told me:

> *For a long time, I made an emotional investment in hope, only to be continually disappointed. Then I made a shift. I accepted that I have this, and would have to live around it. I decided to start writing. All my energy had been going toward feeling better. I stopped investing in that, and started finding ways to invest in my projects. My joy is in words.*

The joy in her words was evident in *Seabiscuit*, which turned out to be a universally praised and beautifully written book.

Be Your Own Advocate and Case Manager

One of the hardest things to accept is that when you are feeling your worst, in some ways, you have to be your best—at managing your health situation. It's rare that a patient will have a physician who functions as advocate and case manager, organizing and arranging the various members of the health-care team and coordinating nonmedical services and approaches. That job most often will fall to you, or if you are particularly lucky, to a spouse, partner, friend, or relative who is your advocate.

But you will need to have someone overseeing and managing your health situation, to ensure that everyone has the needed information and that everyone is working together in your best interest.

Patient empowerment expert and best-selling author Marie Savard, M.D., has some rules about how to be your own advocate and manager, and get the best possible outcome:

1. Trust your instincts. You are the best expert on you!
2. Collect, read, and organize *all* your medical information, making it available to every practitioner you see who needs it.
3. Research your condition/symptoms, do your homework on you, so you truly can learn as much, if not more than, your practitioner about your condition.
4. Form an active partnership with all your practitioners, which means both sides have obligations to each other and respect each other.
5. Share in all the decisions about your care and treatment.
6. Find the courage to treat yourself right! Once you know the right course for you, stick to it.

Part of being your own advocate is putting yourself first, as Joanne describes it:

Because FMS is invisible (people cannot visually see your disability or see your pain) someone who suffers from this must learn to put himself or herself first, even if it means saying "no" to someone else. If the person is a friend, he'll understand; if not, it doesn't matter. You have to be good to yourself, first, or you'll be no good to anyone. If anything, this syndrome can be enlightening in that you finally learn that being selfish is not always a bad thing. No one will love you and care for you more than you care for yourself.

Get Organized

It's very important to be as organized as possible about your health information. Consider keeping a binder, computer file, or other type of log that includes medical history, test results, files, records, practitioner information, prescription and supplement information, and other details that will be of help to you and your various practitioners.

As discussed in the chapter on finding and working with doctors, it's essential to be organized, and prepared for even your initial visits with practitioners.

Brain fog, "fibro-fog," and memory problems can complicate your interactions, so avoid complications and confusion by asking for written instructions and drug information. Make an audiotape of doctor's visits, with your practitioner's permission, if you need to for backup and review of information.

Put Together a Terrific Practitioner Team

Don't underestimate how essential it is to have the right practitioners on your team. As described in the previous chapter, you need to select carefully the people who will be your partners and guides in the search for better health and the selection of treatments for your CFS or fibromyalgia.

Reduce Stress

There is no question that stress—both physical and mental—can negatively affect the CFS/fibromyalgia process and become an impediment to feeling well. Research has shown that stress causes an immune system shift to a Th2-type response, which exacerbates the chronic nature of conditions such as CFS and fibromyalgia— symptoms seem to flare up and calm down in some people. Stress and emotions can affect our immune system. Neuroimmunologists have mapped how brain cells communicate with immune cells, elevating or calming down the body's response to stress. Relaxation and stress-reduction techniques enhance your immune system and enhance healing, so an essential part of your plan needs to be a stress-reduction approach that works for you.

Incorporate Mind–Body Wellness into Your Program

Whether it's organized religion or prayer, or nonreligious activities such as meditation, tai chi, breathing therapy, or Pilates, mind–body approaches can put your mind and spirit into communication with your immune system. Incorporating some sort of mind–body approach into your plan can greatly enhance immunity.

Optimize Sleep

Sleep is a basic foundation of a successful immune system. Two people can be in a similar state of health, but if one is getting insufficient sleep—and for most Americans that means less than eight hours a night—he or she will have reduced immunity to disease.

Despite what you may think, you cannot become accustomed to insufficient sleep, or "catch up" on chronic sleep deprivation. One University of Pennsylvania study found that multiple nights of little sleep—fewer than six hours a night—could impair mental performance as much as not sleeping at all for forty-eight hours straight. The study also found that people sleeping less than eight hours a night had slower reaction times, were less able to think clearly, and had impaired memory.

One of your chief objectives in CFS/fibromyalgia treatment should be to optimize your sleep. On your own, as a basic part of your plan, should be using the optimum sleep hygiene techniques outlined in chapter 13.

Take a Good Multivitamin Antioxidant Supplement

Most people can benefit from taking a well-rounded multivitamin antioxidant supplement. This should include all your basic vitamins, the B vitamins, vitamin E, plus minerals like selenium, and other nutrients and antioxidants. This ensures that you are getting at least basic coverage on the key nutrients. To simplify the process, one complete antioxidant that has been specially formulated for CFS and fibromyalgia patients is Dr. Jacob Teitelbaum's Daily Energy Enfusion. It's a powder that you make into a drink and take along with one supplement capsule, which replaces as many as twenty different antioxidant pills and daily supplements.

Dietary Changes

There are a number of other essential dietary changes that everyone should make as part of their basic plan:

• **Increase good fats.** The kind of fat you eat helps to determine the way your body handles inflammation. So you need to incorporate anti-inflammatory, healthy fatty acids into your diet in lieu of bad fats. Avoid polyunsaturated vegetable oils and products made from them, including margarine. Avoid the most fatty cuts of meat and high-fat baked goods. When you need to use oils, use olive oil. Fats in your diet should primarily come from lean cuts of meat, poultry, and fish, olive oil, nuts, seeds, and fatty fruits such as avocado and olives.

- **Limit alcohol.** Too much alcohol puts a strain on your immune system, so you don't want to drink to excess. In particular, consider limiting your alcohol intake to red wines, which have some health benefit not necessarily seen in beer and hard liquors.
- **Eliminate or limit caffeine.** Caffeine is an artificial stimulant that puts stress on the immune system and the adrenals. Consider limiting, or even eliminating, your caffeine intake.
- **Eat more vegetables.** One of the things most of us can do to be more healthy is to eat more vegetables. Nutrition guidelines tell us to eat five fruits and vegetables a day, but the reality is that we really should be eating more like nine servings of fruits and vegetables a day, with emphasis on the vegetables.
- **Eat more immune system–enhancing foods.** Every day, aim to eat foods that are specifically immune-enhancing. These foods include garlic, maitake mushrooms, fresh yogurt, miso soup, fresh berries, broccoli, and sea greens like dulse, chlorella, and spirulina. Keep in mind that the brighter, deeper colored the fruit or vegetable, the more phytonutrients it has, and the potential to enhance your immune system.
- **Choose pesticide-free, hormone-free and organic whenever possible.** Pesticides, hormones, and antibiotics in produce, dairy products and meats put a strain on your immune system, diverting it from essential tasks so it can focus on helping purge your body of these toxins. By avoiding these foods, you can reduce the load on your immune system, freeing it up for more important tasks that help you feel and live well.
- **Minimize processed foods.** Focus on fresh whole foods as much as possible, such as fresh vegetables and whole grains, eating as few processed foods as you can manage. This maximizes the nutrients you receive and minimizes the chemicals that are rampant in processed foods.
- **Minimize sugars.** Sugars and high-glycemic carbohydrates such as white bread, white rice, and sugary foods are a stress to the

immune system. Dietwise, it can only help to replace some of the high-glycemic carbohydrates with lower-glycemic versions—for example, replace white bread with a high-fiber sprouted-grain bread or sugary juices with fresh water, or white rice with a high-fiber grain like quinoa or amaranth, or even brown rice. Try to eliminate sugared soft drinks (but don't switch to aspartame-laden diet drinks). Switch to club soda, the sucralose-sweetened diet drinks, or make your own—for example, splash unsweetened lemon or cranberry juice in club soda with stevia (a natural, chemical-free, non-caloric sweetener) or Splenda.

• **Add probiotics.** A high-quality, reliable probiotic supplement is an essential part of everyone's daily healthy diet plan. (The brand I take and particularly like is Enzymatic Therapy's Acidophilus Pearls, a patented formula that requires no refrigeration and delivers billions of live cells.)

• **Calcium/Magnesium Supplement.** Most practitioners agree that for CFS and fibromyalgia patients, it's essential to take a calcium and magnesium supplement, ideally at night, when it can help with sleep. The supplement should be in the 1,000–1,500 mg range.

Stop Smoking

There's no need to list all the reasons why you should stop smoking, because you know them. Not only is there the dramatically increased cancer risk, but smoking is a strain on your immune system, and can have a negative impact on your metabolism, often the very thing that you need to be functioning at its best in order to live optimally with CFS and fibromyalgia. Smoking may feel like an energy booster, or you may wonder how you could possibly cope with stopping smoking on top of everything else you have to cope with, but the longer-term payoff is great.

Don't try to go it alone. I stopped after nearly a twenty-year smoking habit, and I can tell you, it can be tough for a hard-core smoker. What helped me was a combination of antianxiety drugs and finding the right activity to trigger my relaxation response—in my case, it was repetitive needlework, including crocheting blankets and embroidering. But you may need a support group, nicotine gum, patches or lozenges, an antidepressant, antianxiety drugs, hypnosis, or other means of help. Get whatever help you need to stop.

Get as Much Regular Gentle Exercise as Possible

Regular physical activity can enhance the immune system, help with sleep, and help with depression and mood. However, not everyone with CFS and fibromyalgia can exercise. But to the extent possible, some sort of activity or exercise, even a few minutes a day of the gentlest activity, should be an objective for all but the most debilitated patients. Even chair exercises or passive stretching in bed can help. A key consideration, however, is that exercise should always be done only "to tolerance," and should not cause postexertional fatigue. If there is fatigue or discomfort after exercise, then you've pushed too hard and need to reduce the level of exertion.

Learn How to Conserve and Manage Energy

The concept of pacing—conserving and managing energy and time—is an essential component of every CFS/fibromyalgia patient plan.

When people with CFS or fibromyalgia have good days, or even start to notice some improvement and signs of recovery, there's a common tendency to try to do as much as possible in terms of tasks, responsibilities, and enjoyable activities. People want to use up the extra energy on long-delayed activities. This push to accomplish many things can actually cause a setback and energy crash, and sometimes even a relapse. This is why learning how to pace activities and conserve energy is particularly important.

Key skills to acquire include time management, how to conserve physical energy in performing daily tasks, body mechanics, appropriate use of assistive devices, and how to break up activities into smaller tasks over time.

Dr. Jacob Teitelbaum, himself a recovered CFS sufferer, says he "has to keep listening to his body for signs of overdoing it.

> *If I overcook my body, it will let me know, and that's a good thing . . . it's good to have a biofeedback tool in your body that warns you when your life isn't healthy. In that way, the disease isn't an enemy, it becomes a teaching tool.*

Join the Organizations

Staying informed about the latest developments and supporting research into new approaches and developments are important parts of your plan. I found the publications, newsletters, magazines, and Web sites of such groups as the Arthritis Foundation, CFIDS Association of America, Fibromyalgia Network, Myalgic Encephalomyelitis Society of America, National CFIDS Foundation, National Fibromyalgia Association, National Fibromyalgia Partnership, National Fibromyalgia Research Association, and many others of tremendous help in researching this book.

These are just a few of the many worthwhile organizations you can join as a key part of your wellness plan. Contact information for many of these organizations is listed in the Resources section of this book.

Lynne Matallana, who serves as director of the National Fibromyalgia Association, describes one important role of a national organization and how it can help. Says Matallana:

> *When it comes to fibromyalgia, most everything that has been advanced has come from a patient organization, in terms of information to the media, to support groups, even to medical professionals. We continue to act as a facilitator of information, because the doctors who are doing the research are often*

so involved with what they are doing that they don't even have time to talk to the other doctors. Media often look at the illness from the "sexy" or "scandalous" aspect of this illness. We're trying to build credibility and present the research to the public in a way that's important, so people can understand and have an interest in it.

Continue Your Education

An essential part of your plan is to stay as educated as possible about your condition. New developments are happening all the time in the area of CFS and fibromyalgia research. Joining the organizations can help, in that many CFS and fibromyalgia patient organizations utilize magazines, newsletters, Web sites, and conferences to disseminate helpful information. There are also a number of books that offer in-depth information on specialized approaches you may be interested in implementing as part of your plan.

In the Resources section of this book, you'll find numerous organizations, Web sites, books, magazines, and newsletters that provide in-depth information and the latest news about CFS and fibromyalgia.

Get Support

Support can be particularly helpful for some CFS and fibromyalgia patients, and finding some sort of support—family, friends, support groups—should be a part of your plan.

The National Fibromyalgia Association's Lynne Matallana recommends, however, that support start at home. Says Matallana:

Support has to come from your family first. Communicating and establishing a really good relationship with your spouse, partner or family is key, and instrumental in how you are going to feel, and how you're going to emotionally deal with this illness. People also need to realize if you are married or very close to a family member, they are going through this as much as you are. It affects their life as much as yours. Look at how you can support THEM in dealing with this.

While some people come to rely on support groups as family, Matallana believes that they should be viewed more as a temporary place for support:

A place to go to get basic information—for information gathering—you can perhaps make friends, people who you may want to keep in your life, if they're positive and you can share ideas.

Matallana cautions that you consider the personality of the group—whether online or in person—and I can't agree more. As a participant in a variety of chronic illness support forums myself, I can tell you that the nature of some support groups can turn them into hopeless complaint sessions, with little productive discussion. Says Matallana:

I don't like support groups where you just whine, or where they don't have some type of informational program (like handouts or speakers).

Others believe that support groups can provide the critical difference. Dr. Bernie S. Siegel, surgeon and author of the best-selling *Love, Medicine and Miracles*, is a believer in support groups. Says Dr. Siegel:

. . . the key element in all of this probably has to do with group meetings. These are opportunities to get a sharing; a new family; and love. When there is the ability to express all of these feelings, an incredible healing occurs in groups . . .

the group seems to be the unique powerful thing. And again I call it the "care-frontation/loving discipline." This is a group where we are here to change. And that's a powerful part of it I think. . . . If there is an area of your life where you feel as though you need healing, I recommend joining a group with a similar affliction. . . . They're all working on the same issues. The self-esteem, and giving up old sick lifestyles. There's discipline there, and love there.

One patient, Marta, has felt that her Internet support group has been a lifeline:

One of the biggest blessings, aside from my new sense of self as a person who IS, not a person who DOES, is the discovery of one special message board on the Internet. It is where I have made dear friends all around the country who also live with CFS/fibromyalgia. Now "my mission" in life where I can no longer give of myself as before is to encourage and love those who so badly need someone to believe in them, including myself. Although I probably will never meet these people in person I know them in the ways that count. I have their trust and they have mine. Together we say to each other the words we need so much to hear from the world: "I understand."

Finding support can be particularly important for men. While women are far more likely to develop CFS and fibromyalgia, there are many men with these conditions. Unlike women, though, the men tend to be less vocal about the conditions, perhaps because of a reticence to discuss their health publicly or a reluctance to admit that they want or need support. Most of the in-person and online support groups and chats for CFS and fibromyalgia are dominated by women, which can also be awkward for men, who may not want to discuss—or hear about—personal health or sexual function issues in a primarily female group.

Bob Hall, founder of the Men with Fibromyalgia Web site, http://www.menwithfibro.com, wrote in his article at the National Fibromyalgia Association Web site, titled "Fibromyalgia from a Man's Point of View":

> *Men lean towards solving the problem themselves. They are accustomed to "fixing whatever is broken." When they discover they cannot "fix" fibromyalgia and they have to live with it, they undergo the very same feelings women do when they make that final decision to learn to live with FM.*

You can find a number of online and in-person local and national support groups, hotlines, and support communities where you can exchange information and emotional support that can help in coping with your condition. The Resources section contains numerous resources to help in your search for the right support group, as well as books and resources for your caregivers and family members. For men with CFS and fibromyalgia, there are some special resources listed.

Maintain Social Contact

One of the unfortunate effects of CFS and fibromyalgia can be isolation. Because CFS/fibromyalgia patients may be bedridden or have severely limited activities, it is far too easy to become isolated from friends and family. When you have limited energy to reach out or take part in social activities and feel as if you have little to give, how can you maintain social connections? Do your best to stay in touch however you can. And be sure to give back something to your friends.

Betty, a patient, describes the important of friends in her effort to live well:

Another help has been supportive friends. People who still include me. Who make allowances for my strangeness, and still encourage me to do what I can, inviting me to join them even though often I cannot. They don't get it, but how can they? They believe me. They laugh with me, not at me, when I lay on the floor to recover, and just keep chatting.

Sibyl McLendon is a Navajo woman living in the American Southwest, a personal empowerment coach for Circle Of Grace, and author of *The Garden Of The Free Spirit.* She offers these suggestions:

Everyone has something to give! Just by talking to another person, you are giving them the gift of YOU. Every person has value and you are no different. You are not your disease. By making the effort, no matter how small it may be, to connect, no one has to be isolated. If you can use the phone, you can call someone.

If you have a computer and Internet access, the world is available to you. Find a group that interests you, or a support group for your illness. Go into chat rooms for people who have the same limitations as you do. In reality, you are only as isolated as you decide you will be. Be creative in your thinking, and remember, you are just as deserving of this type of help as anyone else.

File for Disability if Needed

Debilitating CFS and fibromyalgia can have a significant impact on your economic situation if you have to cut back on, or stop, work. In most job situations, sick pay eventually runs out. You may not have a disability plan through your employer, or even if you do, you may find it difficult to obtain benefits. Social Security disability can also be a challenge.

In 1999, however, the Social Security Administration (SSA) released a ruling—SSR 99-2p, titled "Evaluating Cases Involving Chronic Fatigue Syndrome (CFS)"—which formally states that CFS is a legitimate medical disorder and can be the basis for a disability finding. Until that point, getting Social Security coverage was hit or miss, since SSA employees often denied CFS claims on the grounds that CFS was not a legitimate condition.

Some key recommendations for filing for disability:

• If you haven't been able to work for a year or you don't expect to be able to work, file a claim now.

• File your SSA disability claim no later than eighteen months after becoming disabled. The rationale is that you'll only receive coverage for up to twelve months prior to the date of your application, plus there is a six-month waiting list. If you want coverage for all the months you were unable to work, eighteen months is the absolute latest point you can still file and have a chance at coverage for the early periods of your medically caused inability to work.

• Be sure to get laboratory and clinical tests that are considered supportive to a conventional CFS/fibromyalgia diagnosis whenever possible.

• Have your own doctor perform disability claims examinations whenever possible, and provide documentation of your disability.

• If at all possible, as soon as you file your claim, hire an attorney who specializes in disability law and has experience handling the cases of people with CFS and fibromyalgia cases. The attorney usually will be paid a fee based on your winning benefits, and can help your claim navigate the system more effectively. According to Scott E. Davis, Esq., a Social Security and long-term disability insurance attorney who works with chronic fatigue patients, "You increase your odds of winning your Social Security Disability case by more than 50% if you are represented by an attorney." California Representative Robert Matsui agrees. In Congressional testimony, he said: "In 2000, 64% of claimants [were] represented by an attorney, but only 40% of those without one, were awarded benefits at the hearing level."

Perhaps the most important advice for anyone planning to file for disability is for both you and your practitioner to communicate regarding your symptoms, and then to "document, document, document!" Be sure that you and your practitioner keep detailed records and documentation regarding the severity of all of your symptoms.

Shari explains why this is so important:

I'm on my third try for disability and am still having to prove myself as I never talked to the doctor about my pain, fatigue, depression and ALL that go with it every time I went there. No proof. So my advice to anyone with any chronic illness is when you visit your doctor, tell him all about your problems you are having with fibromyalgia/CFS, even if you're in there for an earache. And when you visit your doctor and he asks how you are . . . NEVER SAY OK! Always tell them about your other problems. Here I sit with no money, no husband, nowhere to go . . . no insurance. My pills are running out. And I CAN'T work right now. And Social Security says, "YOU HAVE NO PROOF!" So always make sure you really talk to your doctor and that your doctor understands and believes in you and your condition.

Consider Where You Live

One important part of your plan is to consider, even if it's not something you can immediately act on, where you live. One survey found that 66 percent of fibromyalgia patients feel that they are significantly affected by weather changes; 78 percent preferred warm weather and 79 percent believed that cold weather made them feel worse. If you have a substantially improved quality of life during warmer months, it may be worthwhile to start planning now to relocate to a climate that is warmer year-round, if at all possible.

Laugh

The physiological response of laughter is the opposite of stress. Research has shown that laughing lowers blood pressure, reduces stress hormones, and boosts immune function by raising levels of infection-fighting cells and disease-fighting proteins. Laughter can also trigger the release of endorphins, the body's natural painkillers, and produces a general sense of well-being.

You may remember Norman Cousins, author of *Anatomy of an Illness,* who became famous as the patient who "laughed away" a near-fatal illness. What Cousins discovered is definitely a factor in good immune health, and however you do it—seeing funny television programs or films, reading humorous books, being around someone who makes you laugh—you need to incorporate laughter into your basic plan.

■ Planning with Your Practitioner

The other key aspect of your plan involves things you need to work with your practitioner to decide. Because these can be essential parts of your ability to live with CFS and fibromyalgia, that only underscores the importance of having the right practitioners and doctors on your team, those who will work as your partners in making the right decisions with you.

Optimize Sleep

Improving sleep is one of the most basic steps you can take with your practitioner. This may involve recommendations regarding herbal support or prescription drugs that can aid in sleep. But ensuring a sufficient quantity (and for most, that will mean at least eight hours) of uninterrupted sleep, including stage 4 delta sleep, is basic to treatment and possible recovery. Your immune system simply cannot heal if you are chronically exhausted or not getting enough of the restorative stage 4 sleep needed to heal the body.

Reduce Fatigue

Reducing fatigue is separate from optimizing sleep, because even though you have optimized your sleep, you may still find yourself fatigued. Here again there are some prescription medications that may be of help or herbal aids (everything from Siberian ginseng to *Rhodiola rosea* to mate tea, for example) that may help in reducing fatigue and enhancing energy without needlessly stimulating of the adrenal system or taxing the immune system.

Optimize Pain Relief

The plan needs to include specific ideas on how to minimize or eliminate your pain. With your physician, you'll need to look at the various options for pain relief, including supplements, antidepressants, pain medications, injection therapies, physical therapy, manual treatments, and other options, and determine which options to pursue.

Treat Infections

Any underlying infections—such as viruses, mycoplasma, or bacterial infections—that may have triggered your condition, or are contributing to its continuation, worsening, or causing relapses need to be identified and treated by your practitioner. This may involve some of the various tests that were discussed earlier in the book, or it may involve more of an intuitive diagnosis process, where instead of doing lengthy, costly, and invasive testing, certain symptom patterns are interpreted as strongly suggestive of underlying infections that are more common in CFS and fibromyalgia, and a course of treatment prescribed to see if it helps as part of the overall treatment approach.

Treat Hormonal Imbalances

Correcting any imbalances in hormones—including thyroid, adrenaline, testosterone, estrogen, and progesterone—is particularly important to ensuring proper immune functioning and providing an environment for the healing of CFS and fibromyalgia.

Optimize Your Immune System

Depending on what your practitioner recommends, you may pursue prescription or nonprescription treatments to help optimize your immune system. These could range from immunotherapies such as allergy shots, to gamma globulin treatments, to use of supplements such as maitake, inositol, cat's claw, colostrum, sterols, and herbs such as olive leaf extract. But it's particularly important that you work with someone knowledgeable to choose the best immune system enhancers to include in your program.

Treat Mood and Depression

Mood and depression are intricately tied to CFS and fibromylagia. Many patients say that they experience mood problems or depression *because of* the condition itself, but it's a classic chicken-or-egg situation. It doesn't really matter if the depression is worsened by the condition or if it is triggered by the condition. The presence alone warrants treatment, since not treating depression can hinder overall well-being and response to other treatments for CFS and fibromyalgia. Again, antidepressant therapy, or in some cases, herbal supplements, may be recommended to help deal with mood swings or depression in CFS and fibromyalgia.

Plan Carefully for Pregnancy

Having CFS or fibromyalgia does not mean that you can't get pregnant and have a healthy baby. The majority of women with these conditions can bear a child successfully. A primary concern, however, is the medicine you are taking, some of which may be contraindicated in pregnancy, particularly early pregnancy. So you should be particularly careful that you are using a reliable method of birth control until you plan to get pregnant. You should have a preconception appointment with an obstetrician who has expertise working with chronically ill women. Discuss which prescription and over-the-counter medicines and supplements you can continue to take preconception, and which you should stop, and any other changes that you should make prior to becoming pregnant.

Plan on early testing using home tests and/or blood tests with your physician to confirm the pregnancy as soon as possible. At the point that you do become pregnant, you may need to further modify your medications and supplements under to your physician's guidance.

Reports show that women with CFS and fibromyalgia may have fluctuating symptoms during pregnancy, but only a minority report a worsening of symptoms. Many women report feeling better or having less pain and more energy during pregnancy and during breast-feeding.

You may need to plan on extra rest during the pregnancy, and push for your physician to monitor you more carefully, including an early ultrasound, as well as to monitor both you and your baby closely.

Carefully Consider Vaccinations

Some experts advise avoiding any vaccines except for those that are urgently needed. A vaccine is meant to teach the body how to meet and defeat a particular antigen. Conceptually, if an actual infection can activate the immune system, and trigger CFS or fibromyalgia, then it's conceivable that a vaccine may be able to do the same thing. Some vaccinations are thought to shift the Th1/Th2 cytokine balance and induce Th2-type response. Anecdotally, there are concerns about the tetanus, typhoid, influenza, hepatitis B, anthrax, and smallpox vaccines, among others. Hepatitis A, polio, rubella, and the majority of the childhood vaccines apparently are not connected, at least as far as anecdotal information. According to U.K. CFS expert Dr. Charles Shepherd, as many as 60 percent of patients experience some worsening in their fatigue and flulike symptoms after a flu vaccine, for example. Dr. Shepherd does not recommend vaccinations if a patient is

> in the very early stages of CFS, particularly when it obviously follows an infective episode; continuing to experience flu-like symptoms, including sore throat, enlarged glands, fevers, and joint pains; or has previously experienced an adverse reaction to that particular vaccine.

Regular Checks

One thing that is particularly important is to make sure that if you are taking various over-the-counter and prescription medications and supplements, your physician regularly performs blood tests to check for side effects of medications and assess liver toxicity. This is something that isn't always done, and patients can suffer the negative consequences of being on too high a dose of too many different medications for too long.

■ Real Life Plans

While there is no way I can share the many hundreds of e-mails I have received that outline various people's plans, and their thoughts about what works for them, here are just a few highlights that show the diversity of what works for real CFS and fibromyalgia patients. How each patient develops and implements a plan is unique, and the outcomes are also unique. But they are also encouraging.

Nancy has pursued a number of treatments and made various changes in her life to, as she says, "have a higher quality of life while coping with a chronic illness." From Nancy's plan:

1. *Assessed my diet and learned about balanced eating, avoiding too many sugars, processed foods, too much caffeine.*
2. *Lifestyle changes included—early retirement, learning to say "no," finding fun things to do, allowing myself to rest when necessary*
3. *Prescription for a medication (Ambien) that allowed me to sleep after over 10 years of severe insomnia*
4. *Learning about lactose intolerance and food allergies and sensitivities that helped to improve irritable bowel syndrome. Eventually, dicyclomine was prescribed to handle debilitating stomach spasms.*
5. *Self-injections of B12 improve stamina and Klonopin protects my brain and handles whatever anxiety may occur*
    Basically it's important to live as healthy as possible and never push the envelope any more than absolutely necessary.

Frances's plan includes a variety of approaches:

Daily exercise, 2-hour nap at midday, sleep aids that allows me to sleep through the night. NADH, DHEA, Armour Thyroid, supplements for Adrenals and Thyroid have made a marked improvement in my cognitive functioning and ability to combat fatigue. Physical therapy especially ultrasound on stiff muscles allowing them to move more freely, and targeted exercise to improve range of motion. Cranial sacral therapy every 3 weeks, therapeutic massage every 2 weeks, natural foods diet as well as enzymes. I now teach water classes for arthritis exercise. In this way I can still teach, have contact with people struggling with my similar issues and I only have 3 classes a week so I can usually make it to the class.

And Frances has several simple but eloquent principles guiding her success:

Do less and enjoy it more. . . . Accomplish one pleasurable thing each day and that's enough. . . . Enjoy the time you have to read a good novel. . . . Cook something that smells delicious and savor it. . . . Talk or email a friend each day . . .

Joan shared some things that she does to, as she says, "keep myself as functional as possible."

- *TRY to stay within the envelope of my energy.*
- *Never plan two activities for one day.*
- *Read passages from books that inspire me, e.g. anything by Rachel Naomi Remen.*
- *When I cannot concentrate, watch a video that is good news or heart warming. Stressful, suspenseful, sad or desperate stories can permeate my soul and make me feel more hopeless. This boundary breakdown seems to be related to the CFS.*
- *I still try to read the New York Times everyday but I have finally gotten to the point where I don't get frustrated if I can only skim.*
- *Take frequent baths.*
- *Arrange garden flowers in small bouquets.*

Joyce believes that it's important to keep trying new or innovative treatments as part of your plan, but to do so with a new, healthier mind-set.

I do try experimental treatments. I have tried a lot of them. I do not give up on trying them. So, to even do so I need to have some element of belief that it might be possible to do something that will make a substantial improvement. I keep it intellectual. I choose something that makes sense to me. I choose a treatment that logically I think might work, and while I am engaged in it I do not fantasize about how if only it worked then I would be able to do this or that. Instead I go through the treatment, like I have so many times before. I give it an adequate trial, I appraise the results, and I am careful with my emotions. I am careful, if I do start to feel better to appreciate it, use it, but not make zealous conclusions. I need to do that at this point.

After much research on her own, Joanne used Dr. Jacob Teitelbaum's guidelines as a starting point. Says Joanne:

I am now taking nine different vitamin supplements (when I remember to take them!), a prescription sleep aid, and Concerta for the depression. This medicine does give me energy to make it through the day working 40 hours a week. Along with two muscle relaxers to help with the spasms. The key to exercise is low impact aerobic videotapes and stretching exercises. I have learned to pace myself. If I have too much activity on one day I usually pay for it the next. My life has definitely changed since the onset of the illness. I give myself extra time to do everything. Where before all was finished on my "to do" list, now I'm happy just to get started. Stop and smell the roses is my motto!

Melissa describes herself as a "relatively high-functioning fibromyalgia patient," but attributes that success to her current treatments:

*I take 10 mg of Elavil in the evening, have an extremely bal-
anced diet, exercise 4–6 days/week, as well as doing yoga and
getting massage therapy once a month. I am soon to start
acupuncture, and I'm crossing my fingers that it will be helpful too. I have shied away from support groups—I have
found that I am better off by not focusing on the pain, and
more on taking care of myself to decrease it. Plus due to my
age (22), I tend to be looked down upon in groups because it
appears that I have been diagnosed "early," despite the fact
that I've had FM for just as long as some post-menopausal
women. I've found that my current therapies work more in
unison and are not mutually exclusive—each one makes me
feel a little bit better when added, so I'm keeping with the
multi-discipline approach. I feel that I am lucky because not
only can I make a difference in others with chronic pain, but
I also do not know what "normal" feels like and cannot
mourn an active life lost. I've come to recognize my limitations, and although I tend to push myself more than I know I
should, I'm getting better at it.*

■ Online Plan Development

If a multidisciplinary approach sounds like the way you want to
proceed, one way to simplify the process of developing your plan is
with an online assessment program developed by Dr. Jacob Teitelbaum, author of *From Fatigued to Fantastic!*

Based on his own diagnostic and treatment approach, he has
spearheaded the development of two online programs.

The "regular"-version online computer program collects
detailed information (it can take up to three hours to fill in the
information and questions, and you'll need to have some test
results handy).

Based on your information, a complex analysis is performed, based on Dr. Teitelbaum's research. For a fee of less than $200, the program provides

- A lab request form so the tests you choose can be done at your local lab, if needed
- A detailed printout that outlines for you and your physician (based on your history) what is causing your CFS/FMS and which natural and prescription remedies are most likely to help you
- A printout that can serve as your doctor's entire medical record—(except for your doctor's physical examination. This saves your doctor hours of time and allows him or her to effectively treat you—even those of you who are not familiar with the illness.

The "short" program, which costs less than $100, takes about thirty minutes to fill in information. This version does not include the complete medical evaluation and record information, and focuses specifically on just what you need to do to optimally treat your CFS and fibromyalgia. A complete medical record is not created.

While both programs include recommendations for prescription drugs, Dr. Teitelbaum has carefully outlined nonprescription alternatives for most treatments, so you can do the treatment program on your own.

While I already have a fairly comprehensive program for treatment of my own CFS and fibromyalgia symptoms, as well as my underactive thyroid, I tested out the long version of the online program to see what it would come up with, based on my symptom profile and medical history.

The program is fairly simple to use, and created about an eighty-page medical record and detailed recommendations program for me. I was surprised to find that based on a few hours of my answering questions, the program pinpointed a number of issues that had taken several years to uncover as part of my regular medical care, and suggested several treatments that work quite well for me—treatments my doctor and I happened upon more by chance than by design. Basically, had I had this program back in 1995, when I had my major relapse, I might have been able to ward off a few of the declines I experienced and saved myself years of trial and error with different drugs, natural treatments, and approaches.

Luckily, my practitioner and I have gotten to a place where I feel fairly well, and we periodically revisit my plan to modify it, based on how I'm doing. But we could have definitely gotten there far quicker with the use of Dr. Teitelbaum's program. It's certainly an option for those CFS and fibromyalgia patients who feel that a multidisciplinary approach may be the way to go and who are looking for somewhere concrete to start their planning process.

16

Finding Hope

> Lord save us all from old age and broken health and a
> hope tree that has lost the faculty of putting out blossoms.
> —MARK TWAIN

When you're dealing with conditions like CFS and fibromyalgia
that have no clear, demonstrable, or easy cure, you may feel
that it's hard—if not impossible—to muster hope or a positive, yet
realistic, attitude about your health.

But hope is essential. Says Charles Lapp, M.D.:

> . . . I can assure you from experience that pushing and crash-
> ing, denial, depression, and a negative attitude are all formu-
> las for disaster, and I have never seen a patient who practiced
> them and yet recovered.

Despite what you may have heard about CFS and fibromyalgia,
people do recover.

In fact, CFS and fibromyalgia are entirely reversible in some
cases. One researcher, Phil Peterson, M.D., of the University of
Minnesota Medical School, conducted a study of 135 CFS patients,
concluding that

Although it waxes and wanes, [patients] generally head slowly out of the woods with this illness. Recovery is . . . clearly the rule in the majority of patients. . . . This is not an interminable disability. Patients do recover gradually.

One study followed CFS patients in four cities over an eight-year period, contacting them every six months to assess their health status and signs of improvement. At the onset of the CFS, more than 45 percent of the patients reported sore throat, fever, tender lymph nodes, general weakness, and muscle pain. Those who had sudden-onset CFS also reported extensive fatigue and sleep, and more brain fog and depression. Recovery was gauged as negative response to the question "Do you still consider yourself sick with a fatiguing illness?" and a positive response to the question "Have you felt better for the last 4 weeks or more?" Using probability analysis based on the results, the researchers found that the probability of recovery from CFS was 31.4 percent during the first five years of illness and 48.1 percent during the first ten years of illness. Recovery episodes can occur at any time, but were more likely in the early stages of the illness, within twenty-four to forty-eight months.

Children and teenagers can have a particularly good prognosis. Dr. David Bell, in a thirteen-year follow-up of children and teenagers with CFS, found that 80 percent had a satisfactory outcome, though with some persisting symptoms. Only 20 percent remained truly ill, with significant symptoms and limited activities or disability.

The type of onset also has an effect on the prognosis for CFS. A Japanese study found that the prognosis after multidisciplinary treatment for patients with postinfectious CFS was better than for those with noninfectious CFS. Postinfectious CFS patients had physical and mental symptom improvement, and a substantial number were able to return to work. Less symptom improvement was seen in the noninfectious CFS group, and fewer were able to return to work and higher levels of activity.

One practitioner who has tremendous hope for recovery of CFS and fibromyalgia is Dr. Jacob Teitelbaum, who has tested his multidisciplinary protocol with scientific rigor and claims a high rate of recovery among his patients. He documented his multidisciplinary approach in a research study that was reported on in the *Journal of Chronic Fatigue Syndrome* in 2001. Dr. Teitelbaum treated patients, as indicated by symptoms and/or lab testing, for 1) subclinical thyroid, gonadal, and/or adrenal insufficiency, 2) disordered sleep, 3) suspected neurally mediated hypotension (NMH), 4) opportunistic infections, and 5) suspected nutritional deficiencies. Among 38 active patients most of whom met both the criteria for CFS and fibromyalgia, at the final visit, 16 were "much better," 14 "better," 2 "same," 0 "worse," and 1 "much worse." Overall, Dr. Teitelbaum reports that 76 percent of the patients on his multidisciplinary approach show improvement after three months and 90 percent improve after two years.

Patients too regularly report their own recoveries.

Jackie describes her experience:

It has now been almost 5 years since being diagnosed with fibromyalgia, and I can honestly say, I am better. I went from being bedridden, needing help with "everything," to being able [to] clean my house, do laundry, go for walks, enjoy life. I surround myself with positive people, and try to sing, laugh, and go outside everyday. The main thing I believe that is key to our feeling better, stay positive. Even on our worst days, there is hope! Make sure to do things that get you out, have people come visit who will make you laugh, and support you. I wake everyday, and thank God for being here. And knowing, that I was so much worse than I am now. I am not always "better," but I allow myself to be "worse." I take it easy, I rest, I tell people "No." I set limits and boundaries, not just for myself, but also for others. So, here is to good health.

Hannah says she's doing what a lot of people with CFS do when they get better:

I'm going back and reclaiming my life, taking it back from this disease, and am picking up where I left off with things that were important to me, and recovering the things I need and bringing them back into my life. One of my supporters is a clergyman at my church. In a recent sermon, he said, "The things you have done in the past, the things you have loved, are never lost to you. They are still there, they are part of you always." He wasn't aiming those words at me, he didn't know I had CFS when he said them, but I think he was led to say those words both for me and for other people who were present who were dealing with losses. I have recently been seeing that what I have done and loved in the past is still there, and his words brought me to tears. They were (and still are) tears of relief, hope, joy that I'm able to have a meaning-ful life in spite of what has happened to me. I believe that my life will continue to get better (especially since my doctor thinks she can bring me into remission and keep me there), and that the worst of it is behind me. I feel like I have an inner health that isn't related to my body's condition, and that's been a stabilizing force in my life.

Be Realistic
Part of staying hopeful, however, means not walking around with Pollyanna pie-in-the-sky expectations. While it's appropriate

for some people to try new therapies in the hope of improvement, remission, or even recovery, being realistic is essential.

One patient, Joyce, says it well:

Hope plays a role. Hope is complicated. Hope to be able to have a life with meaning, to do more of what I value in life is good. Hope to be able to turn the corner on the disease; hope that the next experimental treatment that I try will make a substantial difference is dangerous. I think this is important to understand. Several friends without chronic conditions have thought that hope that I would be cured was essential. However that kind of hope is a poison that keeps one from living one's life—which is in the here and now. Too many people with CFS devalue their life. They say to themselves this isn't living, I will start living once I have found that cure, then I will get my old life back. It puts you in a very vulnerable position. Once a treatment fails to provide the hoped for cure depression sets in.

In an interview with me, author Laura Hillenbrand shared her focus on staying realistic. She doesn't believe in chasing after every fad or new development, or focusing all her attention on having CFS.

Some people get frustrated with me that I'm not more experimental or wildly adventuresome about seeking out new treatment options. But to me, there is something not human or dignified about living all for one's body. That is why I escape to my writing.

But even in being realistic about her life, Hillenbrand has not given up hope. As she told me, "I have never accepted the concept of never getting better. I pray to God that I get better."

Count Your Blessings

As simplistic as it sounds, finding something positive in your situation, and counting your blessings, can be an important part of living well.

Personal empowerment coach Sibyl McLendon says that no matter how bleak the outlook may be in terms of your illness, you still have blessings in your life every day:

You are alive! That is the biggest blessing of all. I strongly recommend spending time every single day, usually at night before going to sleep, listing the blessings of the day. You are alive, you have a roof over your head, food to eat, and maybe you have people around you who love you. They are safe. Maybe today was a day where you were able to do something that made you feel good, even for a moment. These are all significant blessings.

Concentrating on the good, instead of the bad, can make a huge difference in your day-to-day attitude. I am Navajo, and the traditional Navajo greets every day with a prayer of thanks and an offering, no matter how our physical condition may be. Realize that you are so much more than your physical body. Your spirit is alive and well.

Remember, the past is over, done with and unchangeable, and the future is intangible and unknowable. All we really have is this moment in time. Living in the past or worrying about the future will rob you of now. Do your best to make this moment as good as you can!

Nula, a long-term patient, says that coming to terms with the changes in her life has been difficult but doable:

I am in contact with many people who simply don't make that leap, and have been left trapped inside a sick body. . . . I can't be that person, I can't be a victim . . . that doesn't mean I don't have days when I feel sorry for myself, I do! But I know that they will pass and I am getting better at "pampering" myself through them, and learning to use them as days when I recognize that I have been neglecting myself. My whole philosophy is wrapped around these words . . . "You come to believe what you hear yourself speak" . . .

Cheryl found that after eighteen years of CFS and fibromyalgia, one of her main lessons is that out of the worst thing that happened to her could come the greatest opportunities for personal growth and for helping others:

I am a more spiritual person . . . much closer to my religious beliefs. Because I had to leave my career and live on disability 11 years ago, I have been able to devote my life to developing my creative talents. I write, sew, draw, quilt, crochet . . . as my body allows, of course. My experiences with chronic illness and its accompanying loss is helping me help my husband today as he faces a critical point with his quickly developing chronic illness. It's extremely hard on me, too, but what I've had to deal with gives me the strength to be there for him. (This is the man who married me long after I became ill and disabled.) I have been able to provide some little measure of special comfort to two dear friends who passed away within the last two years because they seemed to appreciate and benefit from my history of pain. Indeed these things make my own pain worthwhile.

Learn Acceptance

Acceptance does not mean giving up hope, it just means that you're changing the way you view things and accepting that life is different.

Elsie Owings expresses this well in this stanza from a poem she wrote about her condition:

> No longer can I be a "human doing."
> I can't be in the fast lane anymore.
> I've slowed my pace, and changed my way of viewing
> Priorities that ruled my life before.

Lynne Matallana, director of the National Fibromyalgia Association, feels that acceptance is an important part of hope. Says Matallana:

> You learn to let go of a lot of your fears and the things you have been taught by society—for example, that your worth is based on your income. Having a purpose in your life can be phenomenally healing . . . that doesn't mean you have to save the world. People need to know that they have worth, no matter how ill they are. I used to be a big skier . . . now, I read, sit by the fire, sit with my dog, and then am part of making the dinner and evenings with my friends. Adapting is very important.

One patient, Sarah, has excellent advice:

> If I have learned anything, I have learned that everyday doesn't have to be wonderful. For me to be "just fine" can be okay some days. I recognize that I will have days that are awful, but knowing that at SOME point there will be a good one.

Hannah struggled with accepting her condition:

> For many of the years I was sick, I denied that I had a chronic illness. I had to spend sometimes 2–3 months at a

time in bed, unable to do much of anything, yet I still denied that I had a chronic illness. That was something for other people. I wasn't like that. I had no idea what was going on in my body, though. I eventually had to give up the denial and start learning to live with it. Learning to live with it is a process that has continued over the years. Every now and then, I've had to stop and take a look at what this disease has done to me, how it has guided my life, limited my life, shut doors, cut me off from people and activities that were important to me. I've also had to look at what it means to me in spiritual terms, because it prevented me from being an over-achieving, type-A person who could have been self-centered and insensitive to the pain in the world around me.

Part of acceptance is realizing that you don't have control over everything. A patient, Jessica, describes a letter she received from a wise friend. Her friend wrote:

"I get the feeling that you feel that there is something you can DO, to CONTROL this . . . but one of the things I am thinking about right now is about a healthy attitude being one of curiosity and gentleness—not thinking you have to change a situation or do something different, but just notice what is happening, being curious about it, and being gentle with yourself about it. Maybe there is more of an organic process going on in the world where change can just flower, and we can learn to be in tune with it if we just notice, instead of trying to take charge of it. . . ."

Personal empowerment coach Sibyl McLendon echoes the advice to positively accept limitations and redefine your roles:

Life is so much more than just what a person can do! Your work is not who you really are. Chronic illnesses are often a way for your spirit, your body and/or your soul of telling you it is time for a significant change. If you can't do what you used to do, accept it and discover what you can do now. Just because you can't do what you used to do does not mean you are useless, or that you can't do anything now. Why would you treat yourself in ways that you would never treat anyone else? If a significant other in your life were in the same situation you would never be that hard on them, so don't be that hard on yourself. Treat yourself gently and with love.

Mary Anne describes her own increasing sense of serenity that comes with being at peace with herself and her condition:

Gradually, through isolated moments of mindfulness, I started to experience a feeling of serenity I had never known before. I was coming to terms with my life as it was right now; not a life on hold but a life in progress. This was my reality and I had to accept it if I was going to heal emotionally. I couldn't control what was happening to my physical body, nor was I responsible for anyone else's anger or frustration over my situation. By forgiving myself and giving up the need to control, I was able to feel more centered in my life. By forgiving others who were unable to accept me as a person with a chronic illness, I was able to let go of the unhappiness and resentment that was holding me back from full emotional recovery. For the first time in my adult life, I was able to experience the simplest pleasures, not doing anything, just sitting, watching the tree branches being tossed by the wind, the sun filtering through the window curtains or rain streaming down the windowpane, neither happy nor sad, just sitting, yet feel-

ing more alive and connected with the world than ever before. Improvement of my physical symptoms has been slow, with more relapses than recoveries, but I'm a little more accepting of my body's limits now. I still have moments of despair and feel the tug of guilt nibbling away in the background, but it hangs around less and I don't react with the same intensity. I'm committed more than ever to being the person I want to be, with or without a disability. Most days, I like what I see.

Colleen is a CFS/fibromyalgia patient who has discovered how much she has gained and learned:

Although I have lost much, I have gained life lessons that will never leave me. I have learned to expect the unexpected, and to truly cherish good friends. I have learned that even in hard times it's always good to smile, and that a good cup of tea can make anyone feel better. I've learned that late night phone conversations make me feel special, and that even friends who live hours away can mean the world. I've learned that doctors can be nice, and they can be mean, and to not take personally what someone says to you just because they don't understand. I've learned that I look pretty with or without makeup. I've learned not to get impatient with the person walking slowly across the street, because for all I know, they might have a chronic illness too. And most importantly, I've learned that one day, I will dance again. Whether it is months or years from now, or in heaven, I will dance again. And until then, I will dance with my heart.

■ Being Healed Versus Being Cured: My Own Journey

For more than eight years, I've been on my own journey—a mission to be cured of my chronic illness. I have Hashimoto's hypothyroidism, an autoimmune disease, and battled serious mononucleosis as a teenager, had a half-year period of chronic fatigue syndrome in my early thirties, and had fibromyalgia for nearly a decade. Down deep in my heart, I've always had the belief that somewhere out there is the right practitioner, endocrinologist, herbalist, alternative therapy or mind–body technique—the one that offers the "cure."

What do I mean by "the cure"? Because when it comes to my condition, at least, there is thyroid hormone replacement therapy, which, according to many doctors, may not be a cure but is all the "treatment" I need for hypothyroidism. And for fibromyalgia, I use sleep medicines, an exercise program, and an antidepressant, among other medications.

But by "cure," I really mean returning to the way I used to feel. Feeling well. Being able to come into contact with a simple cold virus and not having it turn into another three-week battle with a flulike illness. Not being so easily fatigued. A neck that never aches as if someone were stabbing it with an ice pick. Arms and legs that don't tingle and ache. A metabolism that isn't glacially slow.

So I started looking. On my journey I've read hundreds of books, talked to hundreds of practitioners, read thousands of Web sites, answered thousands of e-mails, and seen many specialists, a naturopath, two holistic M.D.'s, and a Reiki practitioner. I've tried herbs, supplements, acupuncture, homeopathic medicine, yoga, meditation, Pilates, and tai chi, among other therapies.

I've talked to seemingly everyone; I've tried seemingly everything.

This certainty that the cure is out there somewhere is what spurred me to start a series of health-related Web sites, to write various health-related books, and to become a patient advocate.

When you're dealing with CFS and fibromyalgia, you're focused on feeling your best and figuring out ways to optimize your health.

But for many of us, we become very certain that somehow, somewhere, there are answers out there that will cure us, that will return us to "normal," that will return us to the way we "used to be" before we developed the health condition that challenges us now.

On our journey we fill ourselves with information—reading books like this, surfing Web sites, scouring newsletters, participating in support groups, exchanging information on bulletin boards, and above all, seeing a seemingly never-ending string of doctors, naturopaths, acupuncturists, herbalists, and other practitioners.

We ask questions: "Is this antidepressant better than the one I'm taking? "Would I feel better on a low-carb diet?" "Does this tingling in my arms mean I could have multiple sclerosis?" "What herb can I take to help with energy?" "How can I stop this dizziness?" There are always more questions than answers. It can become an obsession, this search for the one answer that will solve our problems.

But there's a question we really need to ask and don't: What if we can't be cured?

What if, as much as we want it and work toward it, we can't find the answers?

What if we can't ever go back?

What if the only way we can move is forward?

I have a very dear friend who has a serious, but slowly metastasizing, cancer. This man also has an amazing spirit and energy.

He has turned his struggle into a wide-reaching effort to help other cancer patients. While dealing with his worsening health, he founded a huge national cancer support group, ushered it through the process of receiving official nonprofit status, and populated it with an influential and high-profile board of prominent physicians and experts. At the same time, he became an advocate for end-of-life, pain management, and hospice issues, offering workshops around the country on patient rights in end-of-life issues.

All along, he has never given up looking for the medical answers that may hold a key to successful treatment or prolonging his life.

He has a unique ability to live every moment in the moment, without bemoaning the past or worrying about the future. He reaches out to people, puts them together, and creates amazing connections that are changing the world for his fellow patients. It's awe-inspiring to watch.

He is also an incredibly happy man most days.

Watching how my friend has coped with adversity, I realized that there was an important lesson for me. I need to refocus my own efforts, and instead of simply trying to be cured, I should also focus on being healed.

And they are really two very separate things.

Being healed means:

- Accepting myself as I am, even loving myself as I am, with whatever limitations I currently have, without giving up hope that I can improve—in both mind and body.
- Refusing to live in the past and refusing to worry about the future, but instead, living for now, enjoying this time, now.
- Learning how to value myself for what's really important, my spirit, how I live my life, the people I touch and who touch me, instead of focusing on such superficialities as weight changes, thinning hair, a missing thyroid, not having enough energy to do everything I would like to do, needing more sleep than everyone else, and other perceived imperfections

And above all, finding within the cloud of disease a silver lining, the positive effects that having a disease has had on my life.

If you think about it, there have to be some good things that have come from a long-term battle with health issues. Dear friends you've made in support groups, finally starting to exercise, eating better and caring for your health, or maybe learning how to stick up for yourself and your family with doctors. Or perhaps taking time to slow down a bit and take more time for yourself.

I went through this during the writing of this book as I lost my mother to lung cancer. She had battled and overcome breast cancer in her fifties only to have her doctors discover a lesion on her lung in her early sixties. She was never afraid, and felt that she had no choice but to move forward, even when given a terminal diagnosis. She was an inspiration as she delved into living—changing her diet, exploring alternative remedies, taking conventional chemotherapy and radiation treatments, reinvigorating her already strong sense of spirituality—and had two productive, fairly energetic years filled with life and love and family. And that was *after* being told that she had only months to live.

As I was nearing completion of this book, she slowed down quickly, was hospitalized, recommended for hospice care, and succumbed in a few weeks, dying peacefully at home with her family around her. In a letter months before she died, she wrote to me to say that she wasn't afraid of dying, and she was actually happy and at peace.

My concern is for the people here and now that have to go through the anguish of losing someone, that is very difficult. But there is so much beauty in it and if you think of the positive great things that have occurred in the person's life and how they love and are loved, how can you feel sad?

My mother knew she was not going to be cured, but she was truly healed, and her courage and strength was healing to everyone else around her, even in her last days.

For me, having a lifelong chronic disease has introduced me to so many fascinating and pioneering practitioners, made lifelong friends of many amazing and caring fellow patients, and showed me how to treasure the days and weeks and months when I *do* feel well and to *never* take my health or the health of others for granted. It also prepared me to understand and participate more meaningfully in my mother's final years.

As for my friend, his cancer may not be cured, but with his love of life and people and his refusal to focus on the negative, he is certainly healed in his spirit.

He is constantly moving forward, not looking back.

And he is truly so much happier than so many people I know who enjoy far better health than he does.

Ups and downs in health may always be there for those of us with chronic health conditions, but there's one thing that no pill or practitioner or herb can change, and that's how we choose to live our lives, and whether our health controls us or vice versa.

> People are like stained-glass windows.
> They sparkle and shine when the sun is out,
> but when the darkness sets in, their true beauty
> is revealed only if there is a light from within.
> —ELISABETH KÜBLER-ROSS

RESOURCES

This Book's Website

The latest information about CFS and fibromyalgia, the resources featured in this book, and new developments are featured on this book's Web site: http://www.cfsfibromyalgia.com

Contact the Author

E-mail the author at mshomon@thyroid-info.com or write
Mary Shomon
P.O. Box 0385
Palm Harbor, FL 34682

Testing Resources

Antibody Assay Laboratories
AAL Reference Laboratories, Inc.
1715 E. Wilshire #715
Santa Ana, CA 92705
(800) 522-2611 toll-free
http://www.antibodyassay.com/
A highly recommended lab offering a variety of antibody, pathogen, nutritional, allergy, and immunotoxicology testing services.

Ciguatera Testing

Dr. Yoshitsugi Hokama
Department of Pathology
University of Hawaii at Manoa
Biomedical Science
Room D-105
1960 East-West Road
Honolulu, HI 96822
Physicians Information Line: (808) 956-5464.

Great Smokies Diagnostic Laboratory (GSDL)

63 Zillicoa St.
Asheville, NC 28801
(800) 522-4762 toll-free/(828) 253-0621
(828) 252-9303
http://www.gsdl.com
Nationally renowned lab that performs the famous Comprehensive Digestive Stool Analysis of digestive function, tests for candidiasis, immune function, parasite activity, a Comprehensive Antibody Assessment, nutritional assessments, endocrine assessments, and metabolic measures, among others.

Medical Diagnostic Laboratories

133 Gaither Dr., Ste. C
Mt. Laurel, NJ 08054
(877) 269-0090 toll-free
Fax: (856) 608-1667
E-mail: sales@mdlab.com
http://www.mdlab.com
Recommended by leading researcher Garth L. Nicolson, Ph.D., for sensitive polymer chain reaction (PCR) specialty tests for CFS/fibromyalgia patients. Comprehensive testing for tick-borne diseases, chronic fatigue syndrome, viruses and fungi, and mycoplasma infection.

Chronic Fatigue Syndrome/Fibromyalgia-Related Patient Organizations

United States

Arthritis Foundation
P.O. Box 7669
Atlanta, GA 30357-0669
(800) 283-7800 toll-free
http://www.arthritis.org

A large, national nonprofit organization that supports the more than a hundred types of arthritis and related conditions, including fibromyalgia. Information on FM is available on the Web site and in the Foundation's magazine, *Arthritis Today*, which is included with membership. The site also provides listings of local support groups, a fibromyalgia self-help course, and other services and programs.

CFIDS Association of America
P.O. Box 220398
Charlotte, NC 28222-0398
Toll-free voice mail line (800) 442-3437 toll-free
Resource line: (704) 365-2343
Fax: (704) 365-9755
E-mail: cfids@cfids.org
http://www.cfids.org

The CFIDS Association is the leading national organization dedicated to CFS research, education, advocacy, and patient support. The annual membership fee includes a subscription to both of their excellent quarterly publications, *The CFIDS Chronicle* and *The CFS Research Review*. The Web site offers an abundance of CFIDS-related articles and other information, including archives of past issues of *The CFIDS Chronicle*.

Fibromyalgia Network
P.O. Box 31750
Tucson, AZ 85751

(800) 853-2929 toll-free

http://fmnetnews.com

This organization publishes a quarterly newsletter on CFS/FM and related conditions. The annual subscription fee includes a free list of referrals to health-care providers and support groups for your state (in the U.S. and Canada). Free information is also available on the Web site and toll-free by phone.

Myalgic Encephalomyelitis Society of America

P.O. Box 44402

Shreveport, LA 71134

E-mail: MESocofAmerica@yahoo.com

http://cfids-cab.org/MESA

The M.E. Society of America is a research, information and advocacy group seeking to promote understanding of M.E., which is the preferred name for CFS with this group. One of the organization's main goals is "to see the inaccurate, vague, demeaning word 'fatigue' eliminated not only from names but also from descriptions of the disease and from scientific discussion." The site has some good basic information about CFS/ME that emphasizes the seriousness of the illness as well as some scientific references. It offers an online mailing list called *The American M.E. Review*, which publishes articles, advocacy alerts, and research reviews as they arise.

National CFIDS Foundation

103 Aletha Rd.

Needham, MA 02492

(781) 449-3535

Fax: (781) 449-8606

E-mail: info@ncf-net.org

http://www.ncf-net.org

Founded by two long-time CFIDS activists, this organization's goals are to fund CFIDS-related medical research and to provide information, education, and support to those with CFIDS and related illnesses. Its Web site offers a variety of information, with an emphasis on scientific and clinical research. Members receive a quarterly print newsletter, *The National Forum*.

National Fibromyalgia Association

2238 N. Glassell St., Ste. D
Orange, CA 92865
(714) 921-0150
Fax: (714) 921-6920
E-mail: NFA@fmaware.org
http://fmaware.org
This nonprofit organization was originally founded to promote awareness of fibromyalgia among the media and the public. It now provides extensive FM-related information and education through its Web site, a triannual magazine called *Fibromyalgia Aware* (available for a donation), and medical conferences for both patients and physicians.

National Fibromyalgia Partnership

140 Zinn Way
Linden, VA 22642-5609
(866) 725-4404
Fax: (866) 666-2727
E-mail: mail@fmpartnership.org
http://www.fmpartnership.org
A large nonprofit organization that focuses on the dissemination of high-quality, medically accurate FM information to its membership, health-care professionals, and the public. The Web site is chock-full of FM information. Members receive a subscription to the organization's *Fibromyalgia Frontiers*.

National Fibromyalgia Research Association

P.O. Box 500
Salem, OR 97308
http://www.nfra.net
The NFRA is a nonprofit activist organization dedicated to education, treatment, and finding a cure for fibromyalgia. It funds medical research as well as provides both physician and patient education.

New Jersey Chronic Fatigue Syndrome Association
P.O. Box 841
Chatham, NJ 07928
(973) 635-4361
E-mail:webmaster@njcfsa.org
http://njcfsa.org
A nonprofit organization whose purpose is to support patients, disseminate reliable information, and promote research. It sponsors a wide range of activities, including support groups, a quarterly newsletter, statewide conferences, and more.

The Oregon Fibromyalgia Foundation (OFF)
1221 S.W. Yamhill, Ste. 303
Portland, OR 97205
(503) 892-8811
http://www.myalgia.com
Started in 1995 by fibromyalgia experts Robert Bennett and Sharon Clark, OFF is a nonprofit organization that provides information to fibromyalgia patients through its Web site as well as regular educational meetings in and around Portland.

Canada
   Note: Chronic fatigue syndrome is commonly known as myalgic encephalomyelitis (ME) outside the United States.

The Myalgic Encephalomyelitis Association of Ontario
P.O. Box 84522, 2336 Bloor St. W.
Toronto, Ontario M6S 4Z7, Canada
(416) 222-8820
E-mail: meao-cfs@sympatico.ca
http://www.meao-cfs.on.ca
Provides information and support to those in the Ontario area, including support group listings and referrals to doctors and attorneys.

National ME/FM Action Network

3836 Carling Ave.,
Nepean, Ontario K2K 2Y6, Canada
Phone/Fax: (613) 829-6667
E-mail: ag922@ncf.ca
http://www.mefmaction.net
A Canadian organization dedicated to research, education, advocacy, and support. Members receive a subscription to *Quest*, the organization's bimonthly newsletter.

Outside North America

Note: Chronic fatigue syndrome is commonly known as myalgic encephalomyelitis (ME) outside the United States.

Action for M.E.

P.O. Box 1302
Wells, Somerset BA5 1YE, UK
(0)1749 670799
Fax: (0)1749 672561
E-mail: info@afme.org.uk
http://www.afme.org.uk
Action for M.E. is a national charity campaigning to improve the lives of people with ME in the U.K. Members can access a lending library with books and videos, telephone help lines, support group information, and more.

Alison Hunter Memorial Foundation

P.O. Box 2093
Bowral, NSW, Australia 2576
+61 2 4861 3244
Fax: +61 2 4861 3255
http://www.ahmf.org
A non-profit foundation working with researchers and organizations to advance scientific knowledge and medical care and reduce the impact of ME/CFS in the community. Its Web site provides free access to extensive research information and scientific abstracts.

Asociación Argentina Síndrome de Fatiga Crónica
CC N* 114—Sucursal N* 26 (1426)
Capital Federal, Argentina
Phone/Fax: (5411) 4788-0583
E-mail: ecsi@arbitrio.com.ar
Web site: http://www.arbitrio.com.ar/aasfc.htm

Association Française du Syndrome de Fatigue Chronique et de Fibromyalgie
Résidence Porte de Gand-9, rue du Pont à Raisne
59800, LILLE, France
03-20-74-89-02
E-mail: cfs-spid-asso@nordnet.fr
http://asso.nordnet.fr/cfs-spid

Fatigatio e.V.
P.O. Box 410261
D-53024 Bonn, Germany
+49 (0)228-660233
Fax: +49 (0)228-660687
http://www.fatigatio.de

The ME Association
4 Top Angel
Buckingham Industrial Park,
Buckingham, Buckinghamshire MK18 1TH, UK
01280 818960
Fax: 01280 821602
E-mail: enquiries@meassociation.org.uk
http://www.meassociation.org.uk

The largest UK-based national ME/CFS charity provides education, support, advocacy, and research funding. It offers a telephone information line and educational seminars and programs for medical professionals. Members receive a quarterly newsletter.

ME/CFS Society of NSW Inc.
Royal South Sydney Community Health Complex
Joynton Avenue
Zetland, NSW, Australia 2017
(02) 9662 3488
Fax: (02) 9382 8160
E-mail: mesoc@zip.com.au
http://www.zip.com.au/~mesoc
Australian nonprofit organization that promotes research and advocacy
among the medical community and the public; services include a telephone
support line and a newsletter.

ME/CFS Society (SA) Inc.
G.P.O. Box 383
Adelaide, South Australia 5001
(08) 8410 8929
Fax: (08) 8410 8931
E-mail: sacfs@sacfs.asn.au
http://www.sacfs.asn.au
This nonprofit organization provides education, support, and advocacy
services to the South Australian community. Membership includes a sub-
scription to the organization's quarterly magazine, *Talking Point*.

M.E./Chronic Fatigue Syndrome Society of Victoria
23 Livingstone Close
Burwood, Victoria, Australia 3104
Information and support line: (03) 988 88 798
Fax: (03) 988 88 981
E-mail: mecfs@vicnet.net.au
http://home.vicnet.net.au/~mecfs
A nonprofit organization dedicated to serving the CFS community in Vic-
toria and Tasmania; its Web site includes good information for anyone, but
particularly Australian residents.

ME-vereniging Brussel-Halle-Vilvoorde
Dorp 73
B-3221 Nieuwrode, Belgium
0032-16-57 09 83
Fax: 0032-16-57 09 83

South Australian Youth with ME/CFS
G.P.O. Box 383
Adelaide, South Australia 5001
(08) 8410 8929
Fax: (08) 8410 8931
E-mail: sayme@sayme.org.au
http://www.sayme.org.au
Under the umbrella of the ME/CFS Society in South Australia (a nonprofit organization primarily serving members in the local area), SAYME addresses the special needs of young patients and helps them connect with others who understand what they're going through. The site includes sections on CFS news and information, personal stories, and a creative area where members can submit poetry and artwork.

Verein CFS Schweiz
P.O. Box 403
4142 Muenchenstein 1, Switzerland
Fax: +41 (0)61 4138928
E-mail: verein@verein-cfs.ch
http://www.verein-cfs.ch

CFS/FM-Related Professional Organizations

American Association for CFS
515 Minor Ave., Ste. 18
Seattle, WA 98104
(206) 781-3544
Fax: (206) 749-9052
E-mail:admin@aacfs.org

http://www.aacfs.org
A nonprofit organization of research scientists, physicians, and other medical professionals dedicated to CFS research and patient care. Its Web site includes an extensive bibliography of research on CFS.

American College of Rheumatology
1800 Century Pl., Ste. 250
Atlanta, GA 30345
(404) 633-3777
Fax: (404) 633-1870
E-mail: acr@rheumatology.org
http://rheumatology.org
A professional organization of rheumatologists and associated health professionals concerned with the more than a hundred types of arthritis. Fibromyalgia is among the conditions covered.

International Myopain Society
P.O. Box 690402
San Antonio, TX 78269
(210) 567-4661
Fax: (210) 567-6669
E-mail: russell@uthscsa.edu
http://www.myopain.org
A nonprofit organization for research scientists, physicians, and other health-care professionals interested in exchanging ideas, conducting research, or learning more about soft tissue pain syndromes such as myofascial pain syndrome and fibromyalgia.

Professional and Patient Conferences

The following organizations hold annual or periodic international conferences for physicians, researchers, and/or patients. Check their Web sites or contact them directly for information about events currently on the calendar.

Alison Hunter Memorial Foundation
Web site: http://www.ahmf.org
E-mail: ahmfwebsite@hotmail.com
+61 2 4861 3244

American Association for Chronic Fatigue Syndrome
http://www.aacfs.org
E-mail: info@aacfs.org
(206) 781-3544

American College of Rheumatology
http://rheumatology.org
E-mail: acr@rheumatology.org
Phone: (404) 633-3777

International MYOPAIN Society
http://www.myopain.org
E-mail: russell@uthscsa.edu
(210) 567-4661

National Fibromyalgia Association
http://fmaware.org
E-mail: NFA@fmaware.org
(714) 921-0150

National Fibromyalgia Partnership
http://www.fmpartnership.org
E-mail: mail@fmpartnership.org
(866) 725-4404

Chronic Fatigue Syndrome/
Fibromyalgia-Related Web Sites

Canberra Fibromyalgia and Chronic Fatigue Syndrome Pages
http://www.moira.smith.name/index.html
A comprehensive collection of CFS/FM resources compiled by Australian patient Moira Smith. While the site does include many resources specifically for patients in Australia and New Zealand, it's also chock-full of information for CFS/FM sufferers worldwide, including helpful articles, book extracts, and an abundant collection of links.

Centers for Disease Control CFS Information
http://www.cdc.gov/ncidod/diseases/cfs
On this National Center for Infectious Diseases page on the CDC Web site you'll find basic information about diagnosis and treatment as well as a directory of support groups.

CFIDS/Fibromyalgia Self-Help
http://www.cfidsselfhelp.org
Provides information about the CFIDS/FM Self-Help course, a solution-oriented online class that focuses on practical strategies for coping with common problems of CFIDS, fibromyalgia, and related illnesses. The Web site also includes articles on managing CFS/FM, keys to coping and recovery, and success stories.

The CFIDS/M.E. Information Page
http://www.cfids-me.org/
Created and maintained by well-known patient advocate Mary Schweitzer, this site has a wealth of information on all aspects of CFS/FM, including diagnosis and treatment, medical research and references, advocacy issues, support groups, and much more.

"CFS Days"

http://www.geocities.com/cfsdays

CFS sufferer Bill Jackson created and maintains this site, which has a variety of CFS/FM-related articles.

CFSResearch

http://www.cfsresearch.org

This site provides free access to scientific articles on chronic fatigue syndrome, mycoplasma, chlamydia, and rickettsia that have recently appeared in well-known medical journals. For each article there's an abstract available with a link to the publisher's site.

Chronic Fatigue Syndrome & Fibromyalgia Information Exchange Forum (Co-Cure)

http://www.co-cure.org

Co-Cure has an extensive Web site with a wide variety of CFS/FM information. You can subscribe to its online mailing list, which is an excellent source of breaking news, medical journal abstracts, and various announcements about events and activities taking place in the CFS/FM community. You can also search archives of past articles and posts from the mailing list.

"Chronic Fatigue Unmasked"

http://www.chronicfatigue.org

Dr. Gerald E. Poesnecker's Web site contains extensive excerpts from his book, *Chronic Fatigue Unmasked 2000*. His work emphasizes the relationship between the adrenal gland and CFS/FM, and advocates natural remedies rather than drug therapies. The site also includes information about his healing research centers, which offer in-patient treatment.

Devin Starlanyl's Fibromyalgia & Chronic Myofascial Pain Site

http://www.sover.net/~devstar

This Web site from Devin Starlanyl, author of two popular books on fibromyalgia, has a wealth of information for both patients and doctors, with information on diagnosis, treatment, and a list of FM care providers.

The Fibromyalgia Community
http://fmscommunity.org
This site was developed as an extension of a popular online discussion group, "Fibrom-L Listserv." It includes information about the Listserv; but whether or not you choose to join, the site has some helpful resources about FM and related conditions. You can also subscribe to its online newsletter, which highlights articles of interest to FM sufferers, journal abstracts, and more.

HealthWorld Online
http://www.healthy.net
A for-profit site that offers information on a variety of conditions (including CFS/FM), with a focus on alternative medicine. You'll find many informative CFS/FM-related articles on herbal medicine, homeopathy, mind–body medicine, and more.

Immune*Support.com*
http://Immunesupport.com
This site, run by a for-profit company that sells nutritional supplements, provides a wealth of CFS/FMS resources, with a focus on research and treatment news. It has a huge collection of articles and abstracts, disability information, support group listings, and a message board and chat room. You can subscribe to an online newsletter (which typically focuses on CFS/FM news and information rather than the products they sell) and view the archives of past issues on this site.

InfoMIN (Medical Information Network)
http://www2.rpa.net/~lrandall
This site run by Lois Randall offers information and articles on CFS/FM from a variety of sources, with an emphasis on chronic pain.

Living Well with Chronic Fatigue Syndrome and Fibromyalgia
http://www.cfsfibromyalgia.com
The site for this book features updated resources, links, news, and information of interest to readers.

Majid Ali, M.D.

http://www.majidali.com

The author of the well-known book *The Canary and Chronic Fatigue* hosts this site, which includes a variety of articles that focus on his unique theories about CFS and fibromyalgia.

ME-NET

http://www.me-net.dds.nl

This European site has an international emphasis, with access to research databases and official CFS/ME-related texts from all over the world. It includes the most comprehensive list of international links.

Men with Fibromyalgia

http://www.menwithfibro.com

An excellent resource for men who have fibromyalgia and CFS that features articles of specific interest to men and focused on men's issues.

Metabolic Health

http://www.drlowe.com

On his Web site Dr. John Lowe offers in-depth information in an easy-to-read format, focusing on CFS/FM, thyroid disorders, and more—all of which make up what he terms "metabolic health."

The Pediatric Network for Chronic Fatigue Syndrome, Fibromyalgia, and Orthostatic Intolerance

http://www.pediatricnetwork.org

A Web site and online forum for families and professionals concerned with pediatric chronic fatigue syndrome, fibromyalgia, and forms of orthostatic intolerance such as neurally mediated hypotension and postural orthostatic tachycardia syndrome. The resources section includes extensive information on school success and transition planning for adolescents with chronic illness, special education, parenting, and much more.

Remedyfind

http://www.remedyfind.com

Remedyfind is an independent site where individuals and health-care professionals can rate the effectiveness of different treatments for CFS/FM (and other conditions). It also offers a CFS/FM newsletter and links to related sites.

The Road Back Foundation

http://www.roadback.org

This organization promotes education about the treatment of certain diseases (including CFS and FM) with low doses of antibiotics. The Web site serves as a patient and physician clearinghouse for the exchange and dissemination of information on research and the advances in treatment using such therapy, including an online message board for people who are on antibiotic therapy or are considering beginning it.

Self-Study Modules for Practitioners

http://www.cfids.org/profresources/print-self-study-module.ASP

A resource for learning more about chronic fatigue syndrome (CFS), also known as chronic fatigue and immune dysfunction syndrome (CFIDS) or myalgic encephalopathy (ME), has never been easier. The provider education project, titled "Chronic Fatigue Syndrome: A Diagnostic & Management Challenge," is a collaborative effort of The CFIDS Association of America and the Centers for Disease Control and Prevention (CDC), and is designed to teach health-care providers how to better recognize and manage CFS.

WebMD *Health*

http://my.webmd.com/medical_information/condition_centers/
fibromyalgia

This huge consumer health Web site has a "condition center" dedicated to CFIDS and Fibromyalgia, which includes extensive information on diagnosis, treatment, and up-to-date news articles. They also host a selection of CFS/FM message boards, as well as live chat events with a variety of experts (transcripts are also available on the site).

Finding Doctors and Medical Professionals

AMA Physician Select
http://www.ama-assn.org/aps/amahg.htm
Provides basic professional information on virtually every licensed physician in the United States. Search by physician name or medical specialty.

American Board of Medical Specialties
(866) ASK-ABMS or (847) 491-9091
http://www.abms.org
An organization of twenty-four approved medical specialty boards. Their Web site allows you to get certification information for specific doctors by searching according to specialty and locale.

American College of Rheumatology
http://www.rheumatology.org/directory/geo.asp
If you want to find a rheumatologist in your area, you can check the American College of Rheumatology membership directory (searchable by city, state, and country).

American Holistic Health Association
(714) 779-6152
E-mail: mail@ahha.org
http://ahha.org
Offers a searchable database of over two hundred AHHA practitioners who work in partnership with their patients and encourage a holistic approach to wellness.

Best Doctors
(888) 362-8677 toll-free
E-mail: info@bestdoctors.com
http://www.bestdoctors.com
Offers a fee-based online subscription, which provides searches for leading specialists in the U.S., Canada, and abroad.

CFS & FM Good Doctor List

http://www.co-cure.org/Good-Doc.htm

A listing of doctors who have been recommended by and for CFS/FM patients. The physicians are listed on separate pages by city, state/province, and country.

CFS/FMS Doctor Locator

http://beatcfsandfms.org/html/DocLocator.html

A list of well-known CFS/FM doctors and clinics, with information and tips about how to search for and "interview" a potential new doctor.

Devin Starlanyl's Care Provider List

http://www.sover.net/~devstar/provider.htm

According to the Web site, this list is "an attempt to help people find doctors and other health care providers and supporters who have other FMS and/or CMP [chronic Myofascial Pain] patients whom they have cared for in an appropriate and kindly manner."

Fibromyalgia Network

http://www.fmnetnews.com

The Fibromyalgia Network provides referrals to doctors who diagnose and treat fibromyalgia. This service is free with any purchase from their Web store or by calling them at (800) 853-2929.

Questionable Doctors

http://www.questionabledoctors.org

The consumer advocacy group Public Citizen maintains this database, which contains information on doctors who have been disciplined by state medical boards and federal agencies in the past ten years. It contains data on disciplinary actions taken for medical incompetence, misprescribing drugs, sexual misconduct, criminal convictions, ethical lapses, and other offenses.

WholeHealthMD.com Find A Practitioner
whmdpraclookup.wholehealthpro.com
You can use the database provided by American WholeHealth Networks
on this site to find a complementary alternative medicine practitioner.
Search by practitioner type, technique, and location.

Chiari Malformation Resources

Thomas H. Milhorat, M.D, and Paolo Bolognese, M.D.
North Shore University Hospital
300 Community Drive
Manhasset, NY 11030
(516) 562-3020

World Arnold Chiari Malformation Association
http://www.pressenter.com/~wacma/

Online Forums and Discussion Groups

About.com CFS/FM Forums
http://forums.about.com/ab-chronicfatig/
A popular online forum for discussion of CFS/FM-related topics moderated by About.com's guide to CFS/FM.

Co-Cure Message Board
http://www.co-cure.org/msgboard.htm
A message board for open discussions on issues relevant to chronic fatigue
syndrome, fibromyalgia, and related illnesses.

Delphi Forums
http://forums.delphiforums.com
A number of message boards dedicated to CFS/FM and related issues can
be found at Delphi. You can search for forums by keyword or browse
those listed in the "Health & Wellness" channel. Free registration is
required to read and post messages on the boards.

Fibrohugs
http://www.fibrohugs.com/
A large interactive site for FM sufferers and their families, which includes a variety of chat rooms and forums, as well as member submissions and other FM information.

Fibrom-L Email Discussion Group
http://fmscommunity.org/fibromlhelp.htm
An online moderated discussion list where members share advice and support. Individuals with fibromyalgia, their family members, health-care professionals, and any other interested persons are welcome.

GUAIGROUP
http://www.guaidoc.com/newsgroup.htm
An online support newsgroup for people who use and promote the guaifenesin protocol. The discussion group is sponsored by Dr. R. Paul St. Amand and the Fibromyalgia Treatment Center, Inc.

Immune*Support*.com
This Web site offers a message board devoted to CFS/FM. Board members—whether newly diagnosed or those who have been coping with these conditions for a long time—are invited to share information and support.

iVillage.com
http://www.ivillagehealth.com/boards
The health channel at iVillage offers this popular message board dedicated to fibromyalgia and chronic fatigue syndrome.

The Pediatric Network for Chronic Fatigue Syndrome, Fibromyalgia, and Orthostatic Intolerance
http://www.pediatricnetwork.org
A gathering place where teens, parents, education professionals, and others share ideas about managing these conditions in the schools, the medical community, and at home. You can read and post messages or access extensive information on the Web site.

WebMD *Health*

http://my.webmd.com/condition_center/fms
In addition to a wealth of CFS/FM information on this site, you can access their message boards and join in the discussion with other members of the community.

Pregnancy and CFS/Fibromyalgia

Articles on CFS/FM and Pregnancy:

"Childbearing and CFIDS: Making a Difficult Decision"
Dr. Charles Lapp
http://cfids.org/archives/2000/2000-3-article01.asp

"The Effect of Pregnancy on Fibromyalgia Symptoms"
http://www.partnersagainstpain.com/html/assess/assess.htm?pg=6230&section=assess

"Women with Chronic Fatigue Syndrome: Their Experiences of Pregnancy, Childbirth and Caring for Preschool Children"

Bronwyn Carter and Robyn McGarvie
http://avoca.vicnet.net.au/~mecfs/general/pregnancy.html

Finding Support Groups

Centers for Disease Control and Prevention

http://www.cdc.gov/ncidod/diseases/cfs/support/
A state-by-state listing of support groups as well as a few groups outside the U.S. Also includes information on how to select a support group.

CFIDS Association of America

The CFIDS Association of America maintains state-by-state listings of CFIDS support groups and contacts. For a list of support groups in your area, e-mail your name and mailing address to CFIDS@cfids.org or mail your request to The CFIDS Association of America, Attn: Support Group Info, P.O. Box 220398, Charlotte NC 28222-0398. They also offer online information about how to start your own support group and suggested support group activities on their Web site at http://www.cfids.org/community/support-groups.asp

Immune*Support*.com
http://www.immunesupport.com/supportgroups/
A database of CFS and FM support groups in the United States, searchable by ailment and city/state or ZIP code.

National Fibromyalgia Partnership
The National Fibromyalgia Partnership (NFP) maintains a database of fibromyalgia self-help and support organizations in the United States, Canada, and Mexico. If you would like to obtain a printed list of groups in your area, send an e-mail to FMSUPPLIST@fmpartnership.org and provide your name and postal address, and the state/province and country for which you would like self-help or support group information.

CFS/FM-Related Products

The Cuddle Ewe Company
9444 Deerwood Ln. N.
Maple Grove, MN 55369
(800) 328-9493 toll-free
E-mail: info@cuddleewe.com
http://cuddleewe.com
The Cuddle Ewe Underquilt is a bedding accessory popular among fibromyalgia sufferers for its potential to reduce pain and promote restful sleep. The product has undergone limited clinical testing in a study by FM researcher Dr. I. Jon Russell, M.D. (http://cuddleewe.com/research_thumb.htm). The company has been supportive of FM-related organizations and offers some FM information on their Web site.

Fibromyalgia & Chronic Fatigue Guided Imagery Tape/CD
Health Journeys Guided Imagery Audios
Belleruth Naparstek
http://www.healthjourneys.com
This is a fantastic guided imagery tape, and Belleruth Naparstek offers a number of top-quality imagery programs available at bookstores and online.

Pro Health, Inc.
2040 Alameda Padre Serra, Ste. 101
Santa Barbara, CA 93103
(800) 366-6056 toll-free or (805) 564-3064
E-mail: CustomerService@ProHealthInc.com
http://immunesupport.com
Through its catalog and Web site, the company offers nutritional supplements formulated to reduce the symptoms associated with chronic diseases. Many products are designed specifically for chronic fatigue syndrome and fibromyalgia sufferers. The Web site also offers a wealth of free CFS/FM information.

To Your Health, Inc.
17007 East Colony Dr., Ste. 107
Fountain Hills, AZ 85265
(800) 801-1406 toll-free
http://www.e-tyh.com
TyH (To Your Health) offers a variety of supplements formulated for fibromyalgia, chronic fatigue syndrome, arthritis, and chronic pain. Founded as a catalog house by a fibromyalgia sufferer in 1994, the company now also sells products online through its Web site.

Chronic Fatigue Syndrome/Fibromyalgia-Related Books

All About Fibromyalgia
Daniel J. Wallace, M.D., and Janice Brock Wallace
An informative, up-to-date manual that outlines the current understanding

of the disease as well as the latest drug treatments—all laid out in clear and accessible language.

Alternative Medicine Guide to Chronic Fatigue, Fibromyalgia and Environmental Illness

Burton Goldberg and the Editors of *Alternative Medicine Digest*

In this book twenty-six leading physicians explain the techniques and natural substances that brought complete recovery to their patients.

Alternative Treatments for Fibromyalgia & Chronic Fatigue Syndrome: Insights from Practitioners and Patients

Mari Skelly and Andrea Helm

Compiled by two CFS/FM sufferers, this book contains inspiring stories from patients and their personal testimony about alternative treatments that have worked for them. Includes interviews with twenty-eight experts about how their therapy works and how it can help.

America Exhausted: Breakthrough Treatments of Fatigue and Fibromyalgia

Edward J. Conley, M.D.

As the director of the Fatigue & Fibromyalgia Clinic of Michigan, Dr. Conley has treated thousands of patients with CFS/FM and related conditions. In his book he discusses his treatment program and the role of nutrient and herbal formulations in helping CFS/FM patients restore their health.

Beyond Chaos: One Man's Journey Alongside His Chronically Ill Wife

Gregg Piburn

An inspiring and thought-provoking book that encourages readers, both healthy and ill, to become open, honest, and courageous in dealing with the sensitive and difficult issues surrounding chronic illness. The author shares his experiences and insights with a unique combination of wit and sensitivity.

The Canary and Chronic Fatigue
Majid Ali, M.D.
Dr. Ali describes chronic fatigue syndrome sufferers as human canaries—unique people who tolerate poorly the biologic oxidative stressors of the late twentieth century. His book offers information and guidance about nondrug therapies for CFS; also includes sections on hope, spirituality, and more.

The CFIDS/Fibromyalgia Toolkit : A Practical Self-Help Guide
Bruce F. Campbell, Ph.D.
Even though there is no cure for FM/CFS, there are many things you can do to take charge of your condition and your life. This manual for personal change offers a framework to help you understand your illness better, as well as many practical tools you can use to control symptoms and create a more stable life.

Chronic Fatigue Syndrome: A Treatment Guide
Erica F. Verrillo and Lauren M. Gellman
Written by two CFS patients and compiled from extensive research and surveys of other patients, this book is an A to Z guide to every symptom and treatment of CFS.

Chronic Fatigue Syndrome, Fibromyalgia, and Other Invisible Illnesses: The Comprehensive Guide
Katrina Berne, Ph.D.
An updated and expanded edition of the classic book *Running on Empty*, this edition offers the latest findings on chronic fatigue syndrome, fibromyalgia, and overlapping diseases. It includes the whole range of symptoms and diagnostic techniques, and the treatment and self-care options that are available.

The Chronic Illness Workbook: Strategies and Solutions for Taking Back Your Life
Patricia A. Fennell, M.S.W., C.S.W.-R
A comprehensive guide to navigating the physical, psychological, and social aspects of living with chronic illness. The book takes readers on a

journey of self-discovery, enabling them to recreate themselves and their lives.

A Delicate Balance: Living Successfully With Chronic Illness
Susan Milstrey Wells

This beautifully written book examines all aspects of coping with chronic illness, from working with doctors to making accommodations in the workplace. Includes personal interviews with patients, family members, and caregivers.

Facing & Fighting Fatigue: A Practical Approach
Benjamin H. Natelson, M.D.

A comprehensive reference guide to fatigue, relating to CFS and to other causes. Written by a renowned CFS researcher, this book covers a wide variety of symptoms and possible treatments with a no-nonsense approach.

Fibromyalgia: A Comprehensive Approach: What You Can Do About Chronic Pain and Fatigue
Miryam Ehrlich Williamson

A helpful book written in plain English. The author, a longtime sufferer of FM, covers sleep, pain management, relationships, and provides medical and nonmedical ways of managing fibromyalgia.

Fibromyalgia: The New Integrative Approach: How to Combine the Best of Traditional and Alternative Therapies
Milton Hammerly, M.D.

Since no single perspective offers all the answers to the medical problem of fibromyalgia, Dr. Hammerly provides an integrative approach to FM—based on the judicious combination of treatments from Western medicine combined with the best complementary alternative therapies.

Fibromyalgia : A Handbook for Self Care & Treatment
Janet A. Hulme

Written by a physical therapist whose daughters were diagnosed with fibromyalgia, this comprehensive guide includes various subcategories of symptoms with test and treatment plans for each category. The book guides you in developing a personally tailored program of diet, exercise, and daily routines to help you feel more rested, energetic, and pain-free.

Fibromyalgia: A Leading Expert's Guide to Understanding and Getting Relief from the Pain That Won't Go Away
Don L. Goldenberg, M.D.
This book is a comprehensive guide from an expert in the field, based on more than twenty years of clinical research. Dr. Goldenberg separates fact from fiction and addresses causes, symptoms, medication, and natural remedies, using a patient case history to help illustrate each subject.

Fibromyalgia & Chronic Myofascial Pain: A Survival Manual (Second Edition)
Devin J. Starlanyl and Mary Ellen Copeland
In this comprehensive guide, Devin Starlanyl, a medical professional who specializes in the research and treatment of FM/MPS and who has both conditions, and Mary Ellen Copeland, a writer and FM/MPS patient, discuss all aspects of these disorders. Included in the book is information on the latest medications, tips for bodywork, suggestions for coping and obtaining support, and dealing with the health-care system.

The Fibromyalgia Help Book: Practical Guide to Living Better with Fibromyalgia
Jenny Fransen, R.N., and I. Jon Russell, M.D., Ph.D.
From an expert in the field, a how-to guide that provides FM sufferers with practical tools for effectively managing the illness, all laid out in easily understood language.

The Fibromyalgia Relief Handbook
Chet Cunningham
This book focuses on alternative therapies that can help bring relief to muscle pain, fatigue, and other symptoms. An easy-to-read guide that covers such therapies as acupuncture, therapeutic massage, meditation and relaxation techniques, nutritional supplements, and more.

*From Fatigued to Fantastic!: A Proven Program to Regain
Vibrant Health, Based on a New Scientific Study Showing
Effective Treatment for Chronic Fatigue and Fibromyalgia*
Jacob Teitelbaum, M.D.
An authoritative and comprehensive resource guide for CFS/FM. Based on
his own success in overcoming these syndromes and those of the many
patients treated effectively at his Annapolis, Maryland clinic, Dr. Teitelbaum explores the many factors that may be responsible for these conditions and how to treat them. He provides specific guidelines on diagnosis
and treatment, including the use of natural and pharmacological supplements.

*I Was Poisoned By My Body, The Odyssey of a Doctor Who
Reversed Fibromyalgia, Leaky Gut Syndrome, and Multiple
Chemical Sensitivity—Naturally!*
Gloria Gilbère, N.D., D.A.Hom., Ph.D.
Dr. Gilbère chronicles her challenges stemming from a life-threatening fall
and the resulting drug side effects that she believes led to her fibromyalgia,
chronic fatigue, digestive disorders, food allergies, and other problems. She
outlines what led to her recovery, combining personal experience and scientific research, offering natural solutions to complex disorders.

Inside Fibromyalgia
Mark J. Pellegrino, M.D., illustrated by David Schumick
As a leading fibromyalgia expert and someone who has the condition himself, Dr. Pellegrino offers a complete and compassionate "survivors' guide"
that is well organized and easy to understand.

*Sick and Tired of Feeling Sick and Tired: Living with Invisible
Chronic Illness*
Paul J. Donoghue, Ph.D., and Mary E. Siegel, Ph.D.
This book perfectly describes the anguish of coping with illness that others
can't see and provides understanding and practical guidance for coping.
It's a valuable source of help and comfort to sufferers of invisible illness
and their loved ones.

Speeding Up to Normal: Metabolic Solutions to Fibromyalgia
John C. Lowe, M.D., edited by Jackie G. Yellin
This book offers a complete and fascinating overview of Dr. Lowe's metabolic rehabilitation approach to fibromyalgia and hypometabolism.

Stricken: Voices from the Hidden Epidemic of Chronic Fatigue Syndrome
Edited by Peggy Munson
A powerful collection of essays that covers every aspect of living with chronic fatigue syndrome, this book explores the complex social and political dynamics of the illness through the stories of twenty-nine patients.

What Your Doctor May Not Tell You About Fibromyalgia: The Revolutionary Treatment That Can Reverse the Disease
R. Paul St. Amand, M.D., and Claudia Craig Marek
This book outlines Dr. St. Amand's treatment program, combining diet and exercise recommendations with the use of guaifenesin.

Publications

Arthritis Today

This full-color consumer magazine published by the Arthritis Foundation includes articles and other information about fibromyalgia. A year's subscription (six issues) is $12.95, or you can receive a free one-year subscription when you become an Arthritis Foundation member with a minimum donation of $20. Consult the Web site at http://www.arthritis.org or call them at (800) 283-7800 for more information.

The CFIDS Chronicle

The CFIDS Chronicle is the quarterly publication of the CFIDS Association of America and includes information on every aspect of CFIDS and related illnesses. It's offered free to members, and membership costs $35 per year (Canadian: $45; overseas: $60). Membership also includes a subscription to the quarterly *CFS Research Review*, a supplemental publication targeted toward medical and research professionals. For details or to become a member, visit http://cfids.org or call (704) 365-2343.

Fibromyalgia Aware

The National Fibromyalgia Association published its first issue of this full-color magazine in May 2002. The magazine offers research news, information on treatment and self-management, and includes a supplement for medical professionals. You can receive an annual subscription (three issues) when you make a minimum donation to the NFA of $35 (Canada: $45; overseas: $60). Details are available online (http://fmaware.org) or by calling the office at (714) 921-0150.

Fibromyalgia Frontiers

Fibromyalgia Frontiers is the publication of the National Fibromyalgia Partnership. It focuses on providing medically accurate feature articles that are written by reputable researchers, clinicians, and educators in the field of fibromyalgia. It also includes news, research and treatment updates, reflective pieces by patients, publication reviews, and more. A one-year subscription is included with membership in NFP (North America: $25; overseas: $30). Visit the Web site (http://www.fmpartnership.org) or call (866) 725-4404 for more information or to join.

Fibromyalgia Network

This quarterly newsletter, published by Kristin Thorson of the Fibromyalgia Network, which provides patients and health-care professionals with the latest information on FM, CFS, and related conditions; includes articles on new research discoveries, drug breakthroughs, coping advice, and more. An annual subscription is $25 in the U.S. (Canada: $27; outside North America: $30). Order online at http://fmnetnews.com or by phone at (800) 853-2929.

From Fatigued to Fantastic! Newsetter

CFS/FM specialist Dr. Jacob Teitelbaum, M.D., writes this publication he describes as "A newsletter for moving beyond chronic fatigue and fibromyalgia." It focuses on the latest treatment information and also includes questions and answers, interviews with clinical experts, and other CFS/FM resources. A three-issue subscription (approximately twelve to eighteen months) is $35, or you can order a "revolving subscription," in which $9 is automatically billed to your credit card each time a new issue is printed and mailed. Individual issues are also available at $9 each.

Health Points

To Your Health, Inc. (TyH) publishes this newsletter, which focuses on complementary therapies for fibromyalgia, chronic fatigue syndrome, and chronic pain. A one-year subscription (four issues) is $20 (not available outside the U.S.). Customers who place a $25 order through the TyH catalog or Web site receive *Health Points* free. Subscribe online at http://e-tyh.com or call (800) 801-1406 to subscribe by phone.

HEALTHwatch

Published quarterly by Pro Health, Inc. (Immunesupport.com), this newsletter is chock-full of the latest scientific research, treatment news, medical expert advice, and more. It's offered free, and you can request it by visiting http://www.immunesupport.com/healthwatch or by contacting Customer Service by e-mail (customerservice@prohealthinc.com) or by phone at (800) 366-6056.

Journal of Chronic Fatigue Syndrome

A scholarly medical journal dealing with all aspects of chronic fatigue syndrome, for physicians and research scientists. Visit the publisher's Web site http://www.haworthpressinc.com) for detailed information, or contact Haworth Press by phone at 1-800-HAWORTH.

Journal of Musculoskeletal Pain

A scholarly medical journal covering fibromyalgia, myofascial pain syndrome, and other soft-tissue pain syndromes. Visit the publisher's Web site (http://www.haworthpressinc.com) for detailed information, or contact Haworth Press by phone at 1-800-HAWORTH.

The National Forum

Members of the National CFIDS Foundation ($30 annual dues) receive a free annual subscription to this quarterly publication, which includes medical journal summaries, research news, advice on disability issues, reports of expert medical presentations, and more. Visit the NCF Web site at http://www.ncf-net.org or call (781) 449-3535 for information or to join.

Online Newsletters

A number of online newsletter are available on CFS/FM, all of which provide up-to-date news, symptom and treatment information, coping tips, support resources, and much more. Consult the following Web sites for details about each newsletter and how to subscribe.

The Autoimmune Report
http://www.autoimmunebook.com

The Fibromyalgia Community
http://fmscommunity.org/com.htm

Immune*Support*.com Research and Treatment News
http://www.immunesupport.com/bulletins/

National Fibromyalgia Association
http://fmaware.org/newsletter.htm

Remedyfind Chronic Fatigue Syndrome and Fibromyalgia Newsletters
http://remedyfind.com

Financial Support/Assistance

CFIDS Emergency Relief Services, Inc.
4714 Northwood Lake Dr.
East Northport, AL 35473
E-mail: DocESK@aol.com
http://www.cfidsers.org
Doctor Elaine Katz, a professor totally disabled by CFIDS herself, founded this wonderful nonprofit foundation to help chronic fatigue syndrome sufferers with financial emergencies.

Social Security Disability Programs
(800) 772-1213 toll-free
http://www.ssa.gov/disability
If you're unable to work due to CFS/FM or other health problems, you can use Social Security's Web site or contact them by phone to determine whether you are eligible for benefits, find out how to apply, and get access to a number of informative publications.

Planning/Self-Help

Jacob Teitelbaum's online CFS/fibromyalgia planning program
http://www.endfatigue.com
You can access this program at Dr. Teitelbaum's Web site.

CFIDS/Fibromyalgia Self-Help
http://cfidsselfhelp.org
An excellent site that in addition to many helpful articles, features an online self-help course that runs for eight weeks, is held four times a year, and covers key skills, including how to

- Pace yourself to control the "chronic illness roller coaster"
- Set realistic short-term goals
- Reduce stress
- Manage emotions

- Improve relationships
- Minimize relapses
- Develop your own self-management program

Caregiver Resources

Family Caregiver Alliance
690 Market St., Ste. 600
San Francisco, CA 94104
(415) 434-3388
(800) 445-8106 (in California) toll-free
E-mail: info@caregiver.org
Web site: http://www.caregiver.org
Family Caregiver Alliance supports and assists caregivers of brain-impaired adults through education, research, services, and advocacy. FCA's Clearinghouse covers current medical, social, public policy, and caregiving issues related to brain impairments.

National Family Caregivers Association (NFCA)
10400 Connecticut Ave., #500
Kensington, MD 20895-3944
(800) 896-3650 toll-free
Fax: (301) 942-2302
E-mail: info@nfcacares.org
http://www.nfcacares.org
National Family Caregivers Association is a national charitable organization dedicated to empowering caregivers. It offers educational and information services, support and validation for caregivers, public awareness campaigns, and advocacy. It produces a resource guide for caregivers, a quarterly newsletter, manages the Caregiver to Caregiver Peer Support Network, a national resource referral service, and many other services.

Today's Caregiver Magazine

http://www.caregiver.com/

An excellent resource, in print and online, with supportive information for caregivers providing assistance to people with a variety of conditions.

The Well Spouse Foundation

63 W. Main St., Suite H

Freehold, NJ 07728

(800) 838-0879

E-mail: info@wellspouse.org.

http://www.wellspouse.org

Well Spouse is a national not-for-profit membership organization that gives support to wives, husbands, and partners of the chronically ill and/or disabled. Well Spouse support groups meet monthly. Members can share their thoughts and feelings openly with others facing similar circumstances in a supportive, nonjudgmental environment. WS support groups are also an excellent source for information on a wide range of practical issues facing spousal caregivers. Well Spouse support groups exist or are being formed in many areas of the country.

Recommended Readings for Caregivers

The 36-Hour Day: A Family Guide to Caring for Persons with Alzheimer Disease, Related Dementing Illnesses, and Memory Loss in Later Life

Nancy L. Mace, M.A., and Peter V. Rabins, M.D., M.P.H.

Caregiving: The Spiritual Journey of Love, Loss, and Renewal

Beth Witrogen McLeod

The Comfort of Home: An Illustrated Step-by-Step Guide for Caregivers

Maria M. Meyer with Paula Derr, R.N.

Helping Yourself Help Others: A Book for Caregivers
Rosalynn Carter with Susan K. Golant

Related/Overlapping Issues and Conditions

Associations

American Autoimmune Related Diseases Association, Inc.
http://www.aarda.org

American Environmental Health Foundation
http://www.aehf.com

American Pain Foundation
http://www.painfoundation.org

Irritable Bowel Syndrome Association
http://www.ibsassociation.org

The Lupus Foundation of America
http://www.lupus.org

Lyme Disease Foundation
http://www.lyme.org

Multiple Chemical Sensitivity Survivors
http://www.mcsurvivors.com

National Headache Foundation
http://www.headaches.org

National Sleep Foundation
http://www.sleepfoundation.org

Restless Legs Syndrome Foundation
http://www.rls.org

Thyroid Foundation of America
http://www.allthyroid.org

The TMJ Association (Temporomandibular Joint Disease)
http://tmj.org/

Recommended Web Sites and Newsletters

Autoimmune Disease
http://www.autoimmunebook.com

Sticking Out Our Necks: The Thyroid Disease News Report
http://www.thyroid-info.com/subscribe.htm
Request a free sample issue of the print version by sending a self-addressed, stamped envelop to:
Sticking Out Our Necks: The Thyroid Disease News Report
P.O. Box 0385
Palm Harbor, FL 34682

Thyroid Disease
http://www.thyroid-info.com

Other Helpful Books

The Fat Flush Plan and *The Fat Flush Cookbook*
Ann Louise Gittleman, M.S., C.N.S.
Excellent resources outlining a healthy way to eat for life and optimum energy, weight loss, and good health. Gittleman offers sensible, healthy advice on how to eat low-glycemic and low-carbohydrate.

Herbal Defense: Positioning Yourself to Triumph over Illness and Aging
Robyn Landis with Karta Purkh Singh Khalsa
A comprehensive approach to boosting your immune system and overall health through herbs and food.

Living Well with Autoimmune Disease: What Your Doctor Doesn't Tell You . . . That You Need to Know
Mary J. Shomon
The first book to look at autoimmune diseases as a category of illness, focusing on the symptoms and difficult diagnosis process that affects the estimated fifty million sufferers. Features a detailed risks/symptoms checklist and specific information on conventional and alternative diagnosis and treatment.

Living Well with Hypothyroidism: What Your Doctor Doesn't Tell You . . . That You Need to Know
Mary J. Shomon
A comprehensive conventional and holistic look at the undiagnosed, overlooked, and frequently poorly treated condition hypothyroidism, as well as symptoms that plague sufferers, including weight gain, fatigue, hair loss, depression, pregnancy problems, and more. Features a detailed risks/symptoms checklist.

The Miracle of Natural Hormones (Third Edition) and *Overcoming Arthritis*
David Brownstein, M.D.
Dr. Brownstein is a board-certified family physician and is an innovative and leading alternative medicine practitioner. His books provide in-depth information about using natural hormones for hormone balancing and treating arthritis, in particular using various antibiotic protocols. He is the medical director of the Center for Holistic Medicine in West Bloomfield, Mich.

Natural Highs: Supplements, Nutrition, and Mind–Body Techniques to Help You Feel Good All the Time
Hyla Cass, M.D., and Patrick Holford
An excellent book that looks at the various ways to boost mood, mind, and memory—or calm anxiety—using nutrition, supplements, and various techniques. A good reference for someone who wants in-depth information on everything from Saint-John's-wort, to kava, to SAM-e.

The No-Grain Diet: Conquer Carbohydrate Addiction and Stay Slim for Life
Joseph Mercola, M.D., with Alison Rose Levy
An excellent and innovative take on the low-carbohydrate Atkins approach, focusing on the health benefits of a no-grain, very low carbohydrate, low sugar approach, from the director of the Optimal Wellness Center in Illinois.

The One Earth Herbal Sourcebook: Everything You Need to Know About Chinese, Western, and Ayurvedic Herbal Treatments
Alan Keith Tillotson, Ph.D., A.H.G., D.Ay., et al.
A comprehensive look at natural, herbal and nutritional medicine in an understandable format. A required book for anyone interested in natural medicine.

Three Steps to Happiness! Healing Through Joy
Jacob Teitelbaum, M.D.,
A simple but eloquent book that summarizes some basic principles to keep in mind for healing and happiness.

Why Am I Always So Tired? : Discover How Correcting Your Body's Copper Imbalance Can . . .
Ann Louise Gittleman, M.S., C.N.S.
An excellent book that discusses the role of copper and zinc in chronic fatigue syndrome and other immune dysfunctions.

CFS/FIBROMYALGIA EXPERTS

Majid Ali, M.D.
The Institute of Integrative Medicine, the Institute of Preventive Medicine, and *The Journal of Integrative Medicine*
95 E. Main Street
Denville, NJ 07834
(973) 586-4111
140 West End Ave., Ste. 1H
New York, NY 10023
(212) 873-2444
http://www.majidali.com/new.htm
Professor of medicine at Capital University of Integrative Medicine in Washington, D.C., and author of *The Canary and Chronic Fatigue*.

Lucinda Bateman, M.D.
1002 E. South Temple, Ste. 408
Salt Lake City, UT 84102
(801) 359-7400
Dr. Bateman founded her fatigue consultation clinic and has since evaluated more than 550 patients with unexplained chronic fatigue, both CFS and fibromyalgia. She serves on the board of the American Association of Chronic Fatigue Syndrome (AACFS).

David Bell, M.D.
77 S. Main St.
Lyndonville, NY 14098
(585) 765-2060

A well-known CFS doctor who specializes in pediatrics but also treats adults, he is the author of *A Parent's Guide to CFIDS: How to Be an Advocate for Your Child with Chronic Fatigue Immune Dysfunction*, *The Doctor's Guide to Chronic Fatigue Syndrome: Understanding, Treating, and Living with CFIDS*, and *Faces of CFIDS*.

Robert M. Bennett, M.D., F.R.C.P.

Oregon Health & Sciences University
Arthritis and Rheumatic Diseases
3181 S.W. Sam Jackson Park Rd.
Portland, OR 97239
(503) 494-8637
http://www.ohsuhealth.com
Professor of medicine at Oregon Health & Sciences University, Dr. Bennett is one of the leading fibromyalgia researchers and clinicians. He is currently president of the International Myopain Society and serves on the advisory boards of leading patient organizations.

Hal S. Blatman, M.D.

10653 Techwoods Cir., Ste. 101
Cincinnati, OH 45242
(513) 956-3200
http://www.myofascial-solutions.com
Specializing in treating patients with myofascial pain disorders, Dr. Blatman combines conventional and alternative medicine techniques. He is board certified in occupational and environmental medicine and pain management.

Paul Brown, M.D.

1229 Madison St., Ste. 1460
Seattle, WA 98104
(206) 587-0693
Dr. Brown is a rheumatologist who sees many patients with fibromyalgia. (Note: Dr. Brown's office specifies that he requires a referral from another physician, takes very few new patients, and does not accept insurance.)

Dedra Buchwald, M.D.
Harborview Medical Center
Chronic Fatigue Clinic
325 Ninth Ave.
Seattle, WA 98104
(206) 731-3111
http://depts.washington.edu/uwccer/uwchronic.html
Dr. Buchwald is a world-renowned CFS researcher, noted for her CFS twin study and a number of other research efforts. She is director of the Chronic Fatigue Clinic.

Edward Conley, M.D.
The Fatigue & Fibromyalgia Clinic of Michigan
G3494 Beecher Rd.
Flint, MI 48532
(810) 230-8677
http://www.cfids.com
Dr. Conley is a board-certified family practice physician and director of The Fatigue & Fibromyalgia Clinic of Michigan. He is the author of the popular book *America Exhausted: Breakthrough Treatments of Fatigue and Fibromyalgia.*

Serafina Corsello, M.D., F.A.C.A.M.
119 W. 23rd St., Ste. 400
New York, NY 10011
(212) 727-3600
http://www.corsello.com
Founder of the Corsello Centers for Integrative Medicine, Dr. Corsello focuses on alternative and complementary medicine for a variety of conditions, including chronic fatigue syndrome and fibromyalgia.

Derek Enlander, M.D.
860 Fifth Ave.
New York, NY 10021
(212) 794-2000

http://enlander-com.mycoolinternet.net
An internal medicine physician with a specific interest in CFS/fibromyalgia treatment.

Peng Thim Fan, M.D., F.A.C.P.

12660 Riverside Dr., #200
North Hollywood, CA 91607
(818) 980-7010
Dr. Fan's specialty is rheumatology and he treats many patients with fibromyalgia.

Steve Fanto, M.D.

8300 N. Hayden Rd., Ste. A-102
Scottsdale, AZ 85258
(480) 502-0250
Specializes in pain management and rehabilitation and has worked with many CFS/fibromyalgia patients.

Michael J. Goldberg, M.D., F.A.A.P.

5620 Wilbur Ave., Ste. 318
Tarzana, CA 91356
(818) 343-1010
http://www.neuroimmunedr.com
A well-known researcher and clinician, Dr. Goldberg focuses on pediatric neurological dysfunctions, including autism, ADD/ADHD, and CFIDS. He currently treats children only.

Dale Guyer, M.D.

Advanced Medical Center
836 E. 86th St.
Indianapolis, IN 46240
(317) 580-WELL (9355)
http://daleguyermd.com
A family practitioner and director of the Advanced Medical Center, Dr. Guyer blends conventional medical training with his extensive knowledge

of alternative therapies. He treats a large number of patients with CFS/fibromyalgia.

David C. Klonoff, M.D., F.A.C.P.

1720 El Camino Real, Ste. 130
Burlingame, CA 94010
(650) 697-4345
A leading CFS researcher and clinician, Dr. Klonoff is a contributor to the book *Chronic Fatigue Syndrome: A Comprehensive Guide to Symptoms, Treatments, and Solving the Practical Problems of CFS.*

Charles W. Lapp, M.D.

Hunter-Hopkins Center
10344 Park Rd., Ste. 300
Charlotte, NC 28210
(704) 543-9692
http://www.drlapp.net
One of the most well known specialists in CFS/fibromyalgia, Dr. Lapp has written and lectured widely and is involved with a variety of patient and professional organizations.

Susan Levine, M.D.

889 Lexington Ave.
New York, NY 10021
(212) 472-4816
Board certified in internal medicine and infectious diseases, Dr. Levine specializes in CFS and fibromyalgia.

John C. Lowe, D.C.

Center for Metabolic Health
1800 30th St., Ste. 217-A
Boulder, CO 80301
(303) 413-9100
http://drlowe.com
Dr. Lowe is a researcher and practitioner who focuses on a metabolic

approach to fibromyalgia. He is a board-certified pain management specialist and author of *The Metabolic Treatment of Fibromyalgia*

John McFadden, M.D.

Tupelo Pain Clinic
320 S. Gloster St.
Tupelo, MS 38804
(662) 842-2959
http://www.drmcfadden.com
Dr. McFadden's clinic specializes in fibromyalgia and spine pain.

Michael McNett, M.D.

The Paragon Clinic
4332 N. Elston Ave.
Chicago, IL 60641
(773) 604-5321
http://www.paragonclinic.com
The Paragon Clinic is dedicated to treating fibromyalgia and muscular pain.

Roger G. Mazlen, M.D.

148 Tulip Ave.
Floral Park, NY 11001
(516) 352-9483
http://members.aol.com/rgm1/private/mazlen.htm
An internist and clinical nutritionist specializing in the treatment of chronic fatigue syndrome.

Devin A. Mikles, M.D.

CHOICES Integrative Healthcare of Sedona
2935 Southwest Dr.
Sedona, AZ 86336
(928) 203-4844
http://www.choiceshealthcare.com
A board-certified internist, Dr. Mikles is the medical director of CHOICES.

The clinic provides integrative health and healing services with a focus on preventive medicine and the treatment of chronic illness.

Thomas H. Milhorat, M.D.
North Shore Department of Neurology
300 Community Dr.
Manhasset, NY 11030
(516) 562-3020
Dr. Milhorat is a board-certified neurosurgeon who is considered one of the nation's top surgeons for Chiari malformation in CFS patients.

Benjamin H. Natelson, M.D.
New Jersey Chronic Fatigue Syndrome & Fibromyalgia Center
Clinical Division
University of Medicine and Dentistry of New Jersey
The Doctors Office Center, Ste. 8100
90 Bergen St.
Newark, NJ 07103
(800) 248-8005 toll-free
http://www.umdnj.edu/cfsweb/CFS
Director of the NJ CFS/FM Center and a well-known researcher, Dr. Natelson and his staff provide a multidisciplinary approach to patient care. He is the author of *Facing & Fighting Fatigue: A Practical Approach*

David A. Nye, M.D.
Midelfort Clinic
Luther Hospital, Fifth Floor
1400 Bellinger St.
Eau Claire, WI 54703
(715) 838-1900
A board-certified neurologist with a special interest in fibromyalgia and sleep disorders, Dr. Nye has written frequently on the topic of fibromyalgia and is involved with patient organizations.

Mark J. Pellegrino, M.D.
6651 Frank Ave. NW
North Canton, OH 44720
(330) 498-9865

A specialist in physical medicine and rehabilitation, Dr. Pellegrino is a fibromyalgia sufferer and the author of several books on fibromyalgia.

Daniel L. Peterson, M.D.
Sierra Internal Medicine
865 Tahoe Blvd., Ste. 306
Incline Village, NV 89451
(775) 832-0989

Dr. Peterson was one of the physicians documenting the historic 1985 CFIDS outbreak in Incline Village. He is one of the leading CFS researchers and clinicians.

Richard N. Podell, M.D.
55 Kossuth St.
Somerset, NJ 08873
(732) 565-9224
105 Morris Ave., Ste. 200
Springfield, NJ 07081
(973) 218-9191
http://www.drpodell.org

A leading CFS/fibromyalgia researcher and clinician, Dr. Podell utilizes a variety of conventional and complementary treatments.

Thomas J. Romano, M.D., Ph.D., F.A.C.P., F.A.C.R.
205 N. Fifth St.
Martins Ferry, OH 43935
(740) 633-2449

A well-known fibromyalgia researcher and practicing rheumatologist, Dr. Romano has been a caring advocate for the legitimacy of fibromyalgia. He has written and lectured widely in the fibromyalgia and medical communities.

Michael E. Rosenbaum, M.D.

300 Tamal Plaza, Ste. 120

Corte Madera, CA 94925

(415) 927-9450

http://michaelrosenbaummd.com

Specializing in nutritional medicine in the treatment of CFS/fibromyalgia, Dr. Rosenbaum is a co-author with Murray Susser, M.D., of *Solving the Puzzle of Chronic Fatigue Syndrome*.

Russell Rothenberg, M.D.

2141 K St. NW, Ste. 606

Washington, DC 20037

(202) 223-2282

A rheumatologist who specializes in the diagnosis and treatment of fibromyalgia and lupus, Dr. Rothenberg also serves on the board of a leading fibromyalgia patient organization.

Glenn Rothfeld, M.D.

180 Massachusetts Ave., Ste. 303

Arlington, MA 02474

(781) 641-1901

http://wholehealthne.com

Founder and medical director of WholeHealth New England, Dr. Rothfeld is recognized as a leader in the field of integrative medicine and has written and lectured frequently on CFS.

Patricia D. Salvato, M.D.

4126 SouthWest Fwy., Ste. 1700

Houston, TX 77027

(713) 961-7100

A well-known internal medicine practitioner who specializes in CFIDS and AIDS.

Ritchie C. Shoemaker, M.D.

500 Market St.
Pocomoke City, MD 21851
(410) 957-1550
https://www.chronicneurotoxins.com
Dr. Shoemaker, named the Maryland Family Practice Physician of the Year 2000, is the author of a book on chronic neurotoxin-mediated illness, *Desperation Medicine*. Dr. Shoemaker, along with neurotoxicologist H. Kenneth Hudnell, has developed a diagnostic and treatment protocol based on the theory that multisystem illnesses like CFS/fibromyalgia may be caused by exposure to various biotoxins.

David Silver, M.D.

8641 Wilshire Blvd., Ste. 301
Beverly Hills, CA 90211
(310) 657-9650
Currently the clinical chief of rheumatology at Cedars-Sinai Medical Center and assistant professor of medicine at the UCLA School of Medicine, Dr. Silver is the director of the Chronic Pain Rehabilitation Program at Cedars-Sinai.

Stuart L. Silverman, M.D., F.A.C.P., F.A.C.R.

8641 Wilshire Blvd., Ste. 301
Beverly Hills, CA 90211
(310) 358-2234
http://www.drstuartsilverman.com
Dr. Silverman is medical director of the Cedars-Sinai Fibromyalgia Rehabilitation Program, which he founded over ten years ago as one of the first multidisciplinary fibromyalgia programs based on behavioral principles of self-management. He is clinical professor of medicine and rheumatology at the UCLA School of Medicine, and serves on the advisory board of leading patient organizations.

R. Paul St. Amand, M.D.

4560 Admiralty Way, Ste. 355
Marina del Rey, CA 90292
(310) 577-7510
http://www.guaidoc.com

Dr. St. Amand is the pioneer of the guaifenesin protocol for fibromyalgia and author of *What Your Doctor May Not Tell You About Fibromyalgia : The Revolutionary Treatment That Can Reverse the Disease.*

Dr. Roland Staud, M.D.

Internal Medicine and Medical Specialties Clinic
1st floor, Shands Hospital
1600 S.W. Archer Rd.
Gainesville, FL 32610
(352) 265-0139

Associate professor of medicine at the University of Florida in Gainesville, Dr. Staud is a well-known fibromyalgia researcher and practitioner. He is the author of *Fibromyalgia for Dummies.*

Jacob Teitelbaum, M.D.

466 Forelands Rd.
Annapolis, MD 21401
(410) 573-5389
https://endfatigue.com

Dr. Teitelbaum has spent the last more than twenty-five years researching and teaching about effective multidisciplinary therapies for CFS/fibromyalgia. He is the author of *From Fatigued to Fantastic!: A Proven Program to Regain Vibrant Health, Based on a New Scientific Study Showing Effective Treatment for Chronic Fatigue and Fibromyalgia.*

Daniel J. Wallace, M.D.

8737 Beverly Blvd., Ste. 203
Los Angeles, CA 90048
(310) 652-0920

A clinical professor of medicine, UCLA School of Medicine, Dr. Wallace is a leading authority on fibromyalgia and lupus. He is the author with Janice Brock Wallace of *All About Fibromyalgia* and *Fibromyalgia: An Essential Guide for Patients and Their Families*.

Arthur Weinstein, M.D.
Washington Hospital Center
110 Irving St. NW
Washington, DC 20010
(202) 877-0333
Director of rheumatology at the Washington Hospital Center in Washington, D.C., Dr. Weinstein also serves on the medical advisory boards of leading fibromyalgia organizations.

REFERENCES

Chapter 2

Aaron, Leslie A., et al. "Overlapping Conditions Among Patients with Chronic Fatigue Syndrome, Fibromyalgia, and Temporomandibular Disorder." *Archives of Internal Medicine* 160 (January 24, 2000): 201–27.

Afari N., et. al. "Chronic Fatigue in the Offspring of Twins With and Without Chronic Fatigue Syndrome." *Proceedings of the American Association for Chronic Fatigue Syndrome Patient Conference* 2001, abstract #144.

Baumgartner, E., et al. "A Six-Year Prospective Study of a Cohort of Patients with Fibromyalgia." *Annals of the Rheumatic Diseases* 61, no. 7 (2002): 644–45.

Bell, David S., M.D. "Chronic Fatigue Syndrome in Children and Adolescents: A Review," *Focus & Opinion: Pediatrics* 1, no. 5 (1995).

Brehio, Renee. "No More 'Yuppie Flu': New Study debunks CFIDS Myths, Reveals Greater Prevalence." *The CFIDS Chronicle* 12, no. 6 (November/December 1999).

Buchwald, D., et al. "A Chronic Illness Characterized by Fatigue, Neurologic and Immunologic Disorders, and Active Human Herpesvirus Type 6 Infection." *Annals of Internal Medicine* 116 (1992):103–13.

Buchwald, D., et al. "The 'Chronic Active Epstein-Barr Virus Infection' Syndrome and Primary Fibromyalgia." *Arthritis & Rheumatism* 30 (1987): 1132–36, 1987.

Buchwald, D., and Komaroff, A. "Review of Laboratory Findings of Patients with Chronic Fatigue Syndrome." *Review of Infectious Diseases* 13 (1991, Supplement 1): S12–18.

Buchwald, D., et al. "A Twin Study of Chronic Fatigue." Presented at the 5th International AACFS Conference, January 2001.

Buskila, D., et al. "Assessment of Nonarticular Tenderness and Prevalence of Fibromyalgia in Children." *Journal of Rheumatology* 20 (1993): 368–70.

Buskila, D., et al. "Fibromyalgia in Human Immunodeficiency Virus Infection." *Journal of Rheumatology* 17 (1990): 1202–06.

Caro, X. J. "Is There an Immunologic Component to the Fibrositis Syndrome?" In *Rheumatic Disease Clinics of North America*, ed. R. M. Bennett and D. L. Goldberg (Philadelphia: W. B. Saunders Company, 1989), 169–86.

Catton, P. "Treatment Proposed for Chronic Fatigue Syndrome; Research Continues to Compile Data on Disorder." *Journal of the American Medical Association* 20 (1991): 2667–68.

The CFIDS Association of America. "Chronic Fatigue and Immune Dysfunction Syndrome (CFIDS)" Fact Sheet.

DeFreitas, E., Hilliard, B., Cheney, P. R., et al. "Retroviral Sequences Related to Human T-lymphotropic Virus Type II in Patients with Chronic Fatigue Immune Dysfunction Syndrome." *Proceedings of the National Academy of Science* 88 (1991): 2922–26.

"Draft Recommendations of the Name Change Workgroup to be Presented to the DHHS Chronic Fatigue Syndrome Advisory Committee." January 2003. Web site information. Immune*Support*.com.

Forseth, K. O., Gran, J. T., and Husby, G. "A Population Study of the Incidence of Fibromyalgia Among Women Aged 26–55 yr." *The British Journal of Rheumatology* 36 (1997 Dec): 1318–23.

Fukuda, C., et al. "The Chronic Fatigue Syndrome: A Comprehensive Approach to Its Definition and Study." International Chronic Fatigue Syndrome Study Group. *Annals of Internal Medicine* 121 (1994): 953–59.

Goldenberg, D. L. "Fibromyalgia and Its Relation to Chronic Fatigue Syndrome, Viral Illness and Immune Abnormalities." *Journal of Rheumatology* 16 (1989, Supplement 19): 91–93.

Goldstein, J. A. *Chronic Fatigue Syndromes: The Limbic Hypothesis.* New York: Haworth Press, 1993.

Gunn, J. W., Connell, D. B., and Randall, B. "Epidemiology of Chronic Fatigue Syndrome: The Centers for Disease Control Study." *Proceedings of the CIBA Foundation Symposium* 173 (1993): 83–101.

Hader, N., et al. "Altered Interleukin-2 Secretion in Patients with Primary Fibromyalgia Syndrome." *Arthritis & Rheumatism* 34 (1991): 866–72.

Hartz, A. J., et al. "Prognostic Factors for Persons with Idiopathic Chronic Fatigue." *Archives of Family Medicine* 8 no. 6 (November–December 1999): 495–501.

Hoh, David. "Rename It? Debate Centers on Timing, Choices for New Name," *CFIDS Chronicle* 10, no. 3 (Summer 1997).

Jason, Leonard A., et al. "A Community-Based Study of Chronic Fatigue Syndrome." *Archives of Internal Medicine* 159, no. 18 (October 11, 1999).

Klimas, N. G., et al. "Immunologic Abnormalities in Chronic Fatigue Syndrome." *Journal of Clinical Microbiology* 28 (1990): 1403–10.

Landay, A. L., et al. "Chronic Fatigue Syndrome: Clinical Condition Associated with Immune Activation." *Lancet* 338 (1991): 707–12.

Leventhal, L. J., et al. "Fibromyalgia and Parvovirus Infection." *Arthritis and Rheumatism* 34 (1991): 1319–23.

Maupin, Craig. "A Shaky Foundation: Different Illnesses Yet the Same Name? Differences in the Chronic Fatigue Syndrome Community Today." *The CFIDS Report.* March 2003. Web site information: http://www.cfidsreport.com.

Minowa, M., et al. "Descriptive Epidemiology of Chronic Fatigue Syndrome Based on a Nationwide Survey in Japan." *Journal of Epidemiology* 6, no. 2 (June 1996): 75–80.

Moldofsky, H. "Nonrestorative Sleep and Symptoms After a Febrile Illness in Patients with Fibrositis and Chronic Fatigue Syndromes." *Journal of Rheumatology* 16 (1989, Supplement 19): 150–53.

"Names Suggested as Replacements for CFS." *CFIDS Chronicle* 11, no. 1 (January/February 1998).

National Institute of Allergy and Infectious Diseases. "Chronic Fatigue Syndrome." Fact sheet, January 2001.

National Institute of Arthritis and Musculoskeletal and Skin Diseases. "Questions and Answers About Fibromyalgia." Fact sheet, December 1999.

Peter, J.B., and Wallace, D.J. "Abnormal Immune Regulation in Fibromyalgia." Abstracted in *Arthritis & Rheumatism* 31 (1988, Supplement): S24.

Reid, Steven, et al. "Chronic fatigue syndrome." *British Medical Journal* 320 (2000): 292–96.

Reyes, M., et al. "Chronic Fatigue Syndrome Progression and Self-Defined Recovery: Evidence from the CDC Surveillance System." *Journal of Chronic Fatigue Syndrome* 5, no. 1 (1999).

Russell, I.J., et al. "Abnormal Natural Killer Cell Activity in Fibrositis Syndrome Is Responsive in Vitro to IL-2." Abstracted in *Arthritis and Rheumatism* 31 (1988, Supplement): S24.

Russell, I.J., et al. "Abnormal T Cell Subpopulations in Fibrositis Syndrome." Abstracted in *Arthritis & Rheumatism* 31 (1988, Supplement): S99.

Sigal, L.H. "Summary of the First 100 Patients Seen at a Lyme Disease Referral Center." *American Journal of Medicine* 88 (1990): 577–81.

Stokes, M.J., et al. "Normal Muscle Strength and Fatigability in Effort Syndromes." *British Medical Journal* 297 (1988): 1014–17.

U.S. Department of Health and Human Services. "CFS Demographics." Centers for Disease Control report, February 2002.

U.S. Department of Health and Human Services. "CFS Definition." Centers for Disease Control report, February 2002.

U.S. Department of Health and Human Services. "CFS Information." Centers for Disease Control report, February 2002.

Wallace, D.J., et al. "Fibromyalgia, Cytokines, Fatigue Syndromes and Immune Regulation." In *Advances in Pain Research and Therapy* 17, ed. J.R. Fricton and E. Awad (New York: Raven Press, 1990), 217–87.

Wolfe, F., et al. "The American College of Rheumatology 1990 Criteria for the Classification of Fibromyalgia: Report of the Multicenter Criteria Committee." *Arthritis & Rheumatism* 33 (1990): 160–72.

Wolfe, F., et al. "The Prevalence and Characteristics of Fibromyalgia in the General Population." *Arthritis & Rheumatism* 38, no. 1 (1995): 19–28.

Yunus, M.B., M.D. "Gender Differences in Fibromyalgia and Other Related Syndromes." *Journal of Gender-Specific Medicine* 5, no. 2 (2002): 42–47.

Yunus, M.B., M.D. "Towards a Model of Pathophysiology of Fibromyalgia." *Journal of Rheumatology* 19 (1992): 846–850.

Yunus, M.B., M.D., and Kalyan-Raman, U.P. "Muscle Biopsy Findings in Primary Fibromyalgia and Other Forms of Nonarticular Rheumatism." In *Rheumatic Disease Clinics of North America*, ed. R.M. Bennett and D.L. Goldenberg (Philadelphia: W.B. Saunders Company, 1989), 115–34.

Yunus, M.B., M.D., et al. "Antinuclear Antibodies and Connective Tissue Disease Features in Primary Fibromyalgia: A Controlled Study." Abstracted in *Arthritis and Rheumatism* 34, no. 5(1991): R12.

Yunus, M.B., M.D., et al. "Primary Fibromyalgia (Fibrositis): Clinical Study of 50 Patients with Matched Normal Controls." *Seminars on Arthritis and Rheumatism* 11 (1981): 151–57.

Yunus, M.B., et al. "Relationship of Clinical Features with Psychologic Status in Primary Fibromyalgia." *Arthritis & Rheumatism* 34 (1991): 15–21.

Chapters 3 and 4

Altemus, M., et al. "Abnormalities in Response to Vasopressin Infusion in Chronic Fatigue Syndrome." *Psychoneuroendocrinology* 26 (2001): 175–88.

Barron, D. F., et al. "Joint Hypermobility Is More Common in Children with Chronic Fatigue Syndrome Than in Healthy Controls." *Journal of Pediatrics* 141, no. 3 (September 2002): 421–25.

DeLuca, John. "Neurocognitive Impairment in CFS." CFIDS Association of America. *The CFS Research Review* 1, no. 3 (Summer 2000).

Fibromyalgia Network. "Fibromyalgia Syndrome (FMS): A Patient's Guide."

Komaroff, A. L., and Buchwald, D. "Symptoms and Signs of Chronic Fatigue Syndrome." *Reviews of Infectious Diseases* 13 (1991, Supplement 1): S8–11.

Nicassio, P. M., et al. "The Contribution of Pain, Reported Sleep Quality, and Depressive Symptoms to Fatigue in Fibromyalgia." *Pain* 100, no. 3 (December 2002): 271–79.

Reyes, M., et al. "Risk Factors for CFS: A Case Control Study." *Journal of Chronic Fatigue Syndrome* 2 (1996): 17–33.

St. Amand, R. Paul, M.D., "The Guaifenisin Protocol," GuaiDoc Web site, http://www.guaidoc.com/GuaiProtocol.htm

The CFIDS Association of America brochure. "Understanding CFIDS." 1995.

The CFIDS Association of America. "Women and CFIDS." Fact sheet.

U.S. Department of Health and Human Services. "Abstracts: Studies of Causes of CFS." Centers for Disease Control report, February 2002.

Chapter 5

Centers for Disease Control, National Center for Infectious Diseases. "Chronic Fatigue: The Revised Case Definition."

Bell, David S., M.D. *The Doctor's Guide to Chronic Fatigue Syndrome: Understanding, Treating and Living with CFIDS*. Cambridge, Mass.: Perseus Publishing, 1995.

De Meirleir, K., et al. "A 37 kDa 2-5A Binding Protein as a Potential Biochemical Marker for Chronic Fatigue Syndrome." *American Journal of Medicine*, 108, no. 2 (February 2000): 99–105.

Komaroff, Anthony L., M.D. "The Physical Basis of CFS." *The CFS Research Review* 1, no. 2 (Spring 2000).

Lapp, Charles W., M.D. "Chronic Fatigue Syndrome Is a Real Disease." *North Carolina Physician* 43, no. 1 (Winter 1992).

Lapp, Charles W., M.D. "The Role of Laboratory Tests in Diagnosis of Chronic Fatigue Syndrome." *The CFS Research Review* 1, no. 1 (Winter 2000).

Nicolson, Garth L., et al. "Evidence for Bacterial and Viral Co-infections in Chronic Fatigue Syndrome Patients." *Journal of Chronic Fatigue Syndrome,* 2002.

Nicolson, Garth L., et al. "High Prevalence of Mycoplasmal Infections in Symptomatic (Chronic Fatigue Syndrome) Family Members of Mycoplasma-Positive Gulf War Illness Patients." *Journal of Chronic Fatigue Syndrome*, 2002.

Nijs, J., et al. "High Prevalence of Mycoplasma Infections Among European Chronic Fatigue Syndrome Patients. Examination of Four Mycoplasma Species in Blood of Chronic Fatigue Syndrome Patients" *FEMS Immunology and Medical Microbiology* 34, no. 3 (November 2002): 209–14.

Plioplys, Sigita, M.D., et al. "Chronic Fatigue Syndrome (Myalgic Encephalopathy)." *Southern Medical Journal* 88, no. 10 (October 1995): 993–1000.

Schwartz, Richard B., et al. "Detection of Intracranial Abnormalities in Patients with Chronic Fatigue Syndrome: Comparison of MR Imaging and SPECT." *American Journal of Roentgenology* 162 (1994): 935–41.

Sharpe, Michael, et al. "ABC of Psychological Medicine: Fatigue." *British Medical Journal* 325 (2002): 480–83.

U.S. Department of Health and Human Services. "Chronic Fatigue Syndrome: State of the Science Conference." *Report of the Chronic Fatigue Syndrome Coordinating Committee*, October 23–24, 2000.

U.S. Department of Health and Human Services. "Diagnosis of CFS." Centers for Disease Control report, February 2002.

U.S. Department of Health and Human Services. "Screening Tests for Detecting Common Exclusionary Conditions." Centers for Disease Control report, February 2002.

Chapter 6

Buchwald D., et al. "Frequency of 'Chronic Active Epstein-Barr' Virus Infection in a General Medical Practice." *Journal of the American Medical Association* 257 (1987): 2303–7.

Cooper, Deborah. "Lone Voice Proponent of Single Cause Theory of Chronic Fatigue Syndrome." Immune*Support*.com News Service, September 25, 2000.

Holmes, G. P., et al. "A Cluster of Patients with a Chronic Mononucleosis-like Syndrome." *Journal of the American Medical Association* 257 (1987): 2297–302.

"Inability of retroviral tests to identify persons with chronic fatigue syndrome." *Morbidity and Mortality Weekly Report* 42 (1993): 183–90.

Jadin, C. L., M.D. "Common Clinical and Biological Windows on CFS and Rickettsial Diseases." *CFS Research*, 1997.

Jadin, C. L., M.D., "The Rickettsial Approach and Treatment of Patients Presenting with CFS, Fibromyalgia, Rheumatoid Arthritis and Neurological Dysfunction." *Proceedings of the Manly Conference*, February 1999, Republic of South Africa.

Komaroff, Anthony, M.D. "The Biology of Chronic Fatigue Syndrome." *American Journal of Medicine* 108(February 2000).

Lerner, A. Martin. "Method for Diagnosing and Alleviating the Symptoms of Chronic Fatigue Syndrome." Abstract. Report of the United States Patent Office, Patent 6,399,622. June 4, 2002.

Martin, W. John, M.D. "Stealth Virus Infection in Chronic Fatigue Syndrome Patients." Center for Complex Infectious Diseases. Web site information. Immune*Support*.com, January 2002. http://www.immune support.com/library/print.cfm?ID=3266

Nicolson, Garth. "The Role of Microorganism Infections in Chronic Illnesses: Support for Antibiotic Regimens" *The CFIDS Chronicle* 12, no. 5 (September/October 1999).

Nijs, J., et. al. "High Prevalence of Mycoplasma Infections Among European Chronic Fatigue Syndrome Patients. Examination of Four Mycoplasma Species in Blood of Chronic Fatigue Syndrome Patients." *FEMS Immunology and Medical Microbiology*, 34, no. 3 (November 2002): 209–14.

Patarca-Montero, Roberto, M.D., et. al. "Immunotherapy of Chronic Fatigue Syndrome: Therapeutic Interventions Aimed at Modulating the Th1/Th2 Cytokine Expression Balance." *Journal of Chronic Fatigue Syndrome* 8, no. 1 (2001).

Ripper, Jill Richelle, M.D. "Candidiasis." *emedicine Journal*, December 2001. www.emedicine.com/aaem/topic90.htm

Sood, Sunil K., M.D. "Food Poisoning." *emedicine Journal*, August 2002. www.emedicine.com/ped/topic795.htm

Straus, S. E., et al. "Persisting Illness and Fatigue in Adults with Evidence of Epstein-Barr Infection." *Annals of Internal Medicine* 102 (1985): 7–16.

U.S. Department of Health and Human Services. "Possible Causes of CFS." Centers for Disease Control report, February 2002.

Chapter 7

Patarca-Montero, Roberto, M.D. "Directions in Immunotherapy." CFIDS Association of America, *CFS Research Review* 2, no. 1 (Winter 2001).

Patarca-Montero, Roberto, M.D., et al. "Immunotherapy of Chronic Fatigue Syndrome: Therapeutic Interventions Aimed at Modulating the Th1/Th2 Cytokine Expression Balance." *Journal of Chronic Fatigue Syndrome* 8, no.1 (2001).

Rosenbaum, Michael E., M.D., et al. "Improved Immune Activation Markers in CFIDS Patients Treated with Thymic Protein A." Unpublished paper.

Shepherd, Charles, M.D. "Is CFS Linked to Vaccinations." CFIDS Association of America, *CFS Research Review* 2, no.1 (Winter 2001).

Smith, Melissa Diane. "Copper Overload: Do You Have It, and What Can you Do About It?" *Let's Live!* March 1999.

U.S. Department of Health and Human Services. "Possible Causes of CFS." Centers for Disease Control report, February 2002.

Vanderhaeghe, Lorna R., and Patrick J.D. Bouic. *The Immune System Cure*. New York: Kensington Publishing, 2000.

Zachrisson, O., et al. "Treatment with Staphylococcus Toxoid in Fibromyalgia/Chronic Fatigue Syndrome: A Randomised Controlled Trial." *European Journal of Pain* 6, no. 6 (December 2002): 455–66.

Chapter 8

Cleare, A.J., et al. "Low-Dose Hydrocortisone in Chronic Fatigue Syndrome: A Randomised Crossover Trial." *Lancet* 353 (February 1999): 455–58.

Crofford, L.J. "The Hypothalamic-Pituitary-Adrenal Stress Axis in Fibromyalgia and Chronic Fatigue Syndrome." *Rheumatology* 57 (1998, Supplement): 67–71.

Demitrack, M.A., et al. "Evidence for Impaired Activation of the Hypothalamic-Pituitary-Adrenal Axis in Patients with Chronic Fatigue Syndrome." *The Journal of Clinical Endocrinology and Metabolism* 73, no. 6 (December 1991): 1224–34.

"Doctors and Researchers Connect Symptoms of CFS with Adrenal Insufficiency." HealthWatch Holiday 2002. Immune*Support*.com, April 9, 2003. http://www.immunesupport.com/library/print.cfm?ID=4492

Gaab, J., et al. "Hypothalamic-Pituitary-Adrenal Axis Reactivity in Chronic Fatigue Syndrome and Health Under Psychological, Physiological, and Pharmacological Stimulation." *Psychosomatic Medicine* 64, no. 6 (November-December 2002): 951–62.

Paiva, E.S., et al. "Impaired Growth Hormone Secretion in Fibromyalgia Patients: Evidence for Augmented Hypothalamic Somatostatin Tone." *Arthritis & Rheumatism* 46, no. 5 (May 2002): 1344–50.

Raber, J. "Detrimental Effects of Chronic Hypothalamic-Pituitary-Adrenal Axis Activation: From Obesity to Memory Deficits." *Molecular Neurobiology* 18, no. 1 (August 1998): 1–22.

Teitelbaum, Jacob, M.D., et al. "Effective Treatment of Severe Chronic Fatigue: A Report of a Series of 64 Patients." *Journal of Musculoskeletal Pain* 3, no. 4 (1995): 91–110.

Teitelbaum, J., et al. "Effective Treatment of Chronic Fatigue Syndrome (CFIDS) & Fibromyalgia (FMS)—A Randomized, Double-Blind, Placebo-Controlled, Intent to Treat Study," *Journal of Chronic Fatigue Syndrome* 8, no. 2 (2001).

U.S. Department of Health and Human Services. "Possible Causes of CFS." Centers for Disease Control report, February 2002.

Chapter 9

"Autonomic Dysfunction in FMS." *Fibromyalgia Network*, Edition 56, January 2002.

"Clinicians Share Experience, Insights at AACFS Meeting," *CFS Research Review* 2, no. 2 (Spring 2001).

Bou-Holaigah, Issam, M.D., et al. "The Relationship Between Neurally Mediated Hypotension and the Chronic Fatigue Syndrome." *Journal of the American Medical Association* 274, no. 12 (September 27, 1995).

Fogoros, Richard N., M.D. "Dysautonomia," About.com Heart Disease Guide. Web site information. http://heartdisease.about.com, 2002.

Goldstein, D. S., et al. "Dysautonomias: Clinical Disorders of the Autonomic Nervous System." *Annals of Internal Medicine* 137, no. 9 (November 5, 2002): 753–63.

Gracely, R. H., et al. "Functional Magnetic Resonance Imaging Evidence of Augmented Pain Processing in Fibromyalgia." *Arthritis & Rheumatism* 46, no. 5 (May 2002): 1333–43.

Graven-Nielsen, T. "Ketamine Reduces Muscle Pain, Temporal Summation, and Referred Pain in Fibormyalgia Patients." *Pain* 85 (2000): 483–91.

Ito, K., et al. "Effects of L-theanine on the Release of Alpha Brain Waves in Human Volunteers." *Nippon Nogeikagaku Kaishi* 72 (1998): 153–57.

Juneja, L. R., et al. "L-theanine—A Unique Amino Acid of Green Tea and Its Relaxation Effect in Humans." *Trends in Food Science & Technology* 10 (1999): 199–204.

Kosek, E. "Sensory Dysfunction in Fibromyalgia Patients with Implications for Pathogenic Mechanisms." *Pain* 68 (1996): 375–83.

Melleegers, M. "Gabapentin for Neuropathic Pain, Systemic Review of Controlled and Uncontrolled Literature." *Clinical Journal of Pain* 17 (2001): 284–95.

Niboyet, J. E. "Effect of Subcutaneous Ketamine on the Pain Level of Patients with Fibromyalgia Syndrome." *Abstracts from the 2002 Annual Meeting of the International Association for the Study of Pain*, August 17–22, 2002.

Pall, Martin L. "Fibromyalgia, Excessive Nitric Oxide/Peroxynitrite and Excessive NMDA Activity." Immune*Support*.com research paper. Web site information. http://molecular.biosciences.wsu.edu/Faculty/pall.html, February 2003.

Papadopoulos, I. "Treatment of Fibromyalgia with Tropisetron, a 5Ht3 Serotonin Antagonist." *Clinical Rheumatology* 19 (January 2000): 6–8.

Rao, M.D., "Monoamine Reuptake and NMDA Antagonist Profile of Milnacipran: A Comparison to Duloxetine." Society for Neuroscience Meeting, November 7, 2002.

Saper, J. "An Open-Label Dose Titration Study of the Efficacy and Tolerability of Tizanidine Hydrochloride Tablets in Prophylaxis of Chronic Daily Headache." *Headache* 41 (2001): 357–68.

Stenson, Jacqueline. "Brain Scans Document Fibromyalgia Pain." *Reuters Health News*, June 17, 2002.

U.S. Department of Health and Human Services. "CFS Treatment." Centers for Disease Control report, February 2002.

U.S. Department of Health and Human Services. "Possible Causes of CFS." Centers for Disease Control report, February 2002.

U.S. Department of Health and Human Services. "Recovery from CFS." Centers for Disease Control report, February 2002.

Vogin, Gary D., M.D. "Pregabalin Information." *ACR 66th Annual Meeting: Abstract 1653*. Presented October 29, 2002.

Walker, Vicki C. "Feeling Faint? What You Need to Know About Orthostatic Intolerance and CFIDS." *The CFIDS Chronicle* 13, no. 4 (Fall 2000).

Zachrisson, O., et al. "Treatment with Staphylococcus Toxoid in Fibromyalgia/Chronic Fatigue Syndrome—A Randomised Controlled Trial." *European Journal of Pain* 6, no. 6 (December 2002): 455–66.

Chapter 10

Arnold, Thomas, M.D. "Ciguatera Toxicity." *emedicine Journal*, April 2002.

Guyer, Dale, M.D. "Pro Health's Healthwatch Treatment Guide 2002." Immune*Support*.com. Web site information. http://www.immunesupport.com/healthwatch/)

Hokama, Yoshitsugi. "Acute Phase Lipids in Sera of Various Diseases: Chronic Fatigue Syndrome, Ciguatera, Hepatitis, and Various Cancer with Antigentic Epitope Resembling Ciguatoxin as Determined with Mab-CTX." Proceedings of the International Symposium on Toxins and Natural Products, November 17, 2002.

LeRoy, Jim. "Management of Chemical Sensitivities in CFIDS." *The CFIDS Chronicle* 10, no. 2 (Spring 1997).

Chapter 11

Bennett, R. M., et al. "A 1 year double-blind placebo-controlled study of guaifenesin in fibromyalgia." *Arthritis & Rheumatism* 39 (1996): S212.

Cox, I.M., et al. "Red Blood Cell Magnesium & Chronic Fatigue Syndrome." *Lancet* 337 (1991): 757–60.

Evengard, B., et al. "Cerebral Spinal Fluid Vitamin B_{12} Deficiency in Chronic Fatigue Syndrome." Abstract. *Proceedings of The American Association for Chronic Fatigue Syndrome Research Conference*, 1996.

"Fish Oil." *Alternative Medicine Review* 7, no. 5 (October 2002): 389–403.

Kuratsune, H., et al. "Brain Regions Involved in Fatigue Sensation: Reduced Acetylcarnitine Uptake into the Brain." *NeuroImage* 17, no. 3 (November 2002): 1256–65.

Lapp, Charles W., M.D. "Using Vitamin B-12 for the Management of CFS." *The CFIDS Chronicle* 12, no. 6 (November/December 1999).

Plioplys, Sigita, M.D., et al. "Chronic Fatigue Syndrome (Myalgic Encephalopathy)." *Southern Medical Journal* 88, no. 10 (October 1995): 993–1000.

Puri, B.K., et al. "Relative Increase in Choline in the Occipital Cortex in Chronic Fatigue Syndrome." *Acta Psychiatrica Scandinavia* 106, no. 3 (September 2002): 224–26.

Romano, T.J., and Stiller, J.W. "Magnesium Deficiency in Fibromyalgia Syndrome." *Journal of Nutritional Medicine* 4 (1994): 165–67.

Seelig, M. "Review and Hypothesis: Might Patients with the Chronic Fatigue Syndrome Have Latent Tetany of Magnesium Deficiency?" *Journal of Chronic Fatigue Syndrome* 4 (1998): 2.

St. Amand, R. Paul, M.D. "The Guaifenisin Protocol," GuaiDoc Web site. http://www.guaidoc.com/GuaiProtocol.htm

St. Amand, R. Paul, M.D. "A Response to the Oregon Study's Implication." *Clinical Bulletin of Myofascial Therapy* 2, no. 4 (1997).

St. Amand, R. Paul, M.D. "Treating Fibromyalgia with Guaifenesin." Immune*Support*.com, October 4, 2001.

St. Amand, R. Paul, M.D., and Marek, Claudia Craig. *What Your Doctor May Not Tell You About Fibromyalgia: The Revolutionary Treatment That Can Reverse the Disease.* New York: Warner Books, 1999.

U.S. Department of Health and Human Services. "Possible Causes of CFS." Centers for Disease Control report, February 2002.

Wagner, Daniel T. "Clinical Versus Alternative Approaches to Treating Fibromyalgia." Doctoral thesis study with survey questionnaire, 2002. www.nauticom.net/www/nutrifrm/fibro.html

Chapter 12

Anderson, Brent D., and Spector, A. "Introduction to Pilates-Based Rehabilitation." *Complementary Medicine*, 1059–1516, 2000.

Bennett, Robert, M.D. *Summary of Abstracts from the 2002 Annual Meeting of the International Association for the Study of Pain*, August 17–22, 2002.

Berman, B.M., et al. "The Evidence for Acupuncture as a Treatment for Rheumatologic Conditions." *Rheumatic Diseases Clinics of North America* 26, no.1 (February 2000): 103–15.

Djuric, Vladimir, M.D. "Treatment for Whiplash, Chronic Neck Pain and Headaches." *Fibromyalgia Network*, October 2000, 51st edition.

Donaldson, S., et al. "Fibromyalgia: A Retrospective Study of 252 Consecutive Referrals." *Canadian Journal of Clinical Medicine 5*, no. 6 (June 1998): 116–27.

Esty, Mary Lee. "EEG Neurotherapy: A Promising New Treatment for FMS?" Presentation to the National Fibromyalgia Partnership, Vienna, Va., June 6, 1998.

Esty, Mary Lee. "Post-Traumatic Fibromyalgia: A New Paradigm." *Fibromyalgia Frontiers* (July/August 1998 and September/October 1999).

Hoh, David. "Spine, Skull Surgery May Help Many with CFIDS, FMS: Chiari Malformation or Squeezing of Spinal Cord May Be Common in CFIDS, Fibromyalgia." *The CFIDS Chronicle*, May/June 1999.

Kelly, Alice Lesch. "Rest for the Weary." *Yoga Journal*, March/April 2001.

King, S.J., et al. "The Effects of Exercise and Education, Individually or Combined, in Women with Fibromyalgia." *Journal of Rheumatology* 29, no. 12 (December 2002): 2620–27.

"Learning to Function With Less Effort, Less Pain." *Fibromyalgia Network*, July 1998.

Mueller, H., et al. "Treatment of Fibromyalgia Incorporating EEG-Driven Stimulation: A Clinical Outcomes Study." *Journal of Clinical Psychology* 57, no. 7 (2001): 933–52.

Neumann, L., et al. "Outcome of posttraumatic fibromyalgia: A 3-year follow-up of 78 cases of cervical spine injuries." Epidemiology Department, Department of Medicine, Soroka Medical Center, Faculty of Health Sciences, Ben-Gurion University of the Negev, Beer Sheva, Israel. *Seminar in Arthritis and Rheumatism*, April 21, 2003; 32(5): 320–25.

"Neurosurgery and CFS: Many Questions Still Remain." *The CFIDS Chronicle* 13, no. 2 (Spring 2000).

Richards, S.C.M., and Scott, D.L. "Prescribed Exercise in People with Fibromyalgia: Parallel Group Randomised Controlled Trial." *British Medical Journal* 325, no. 7357 (July 27, 2002): 185.

Schmidt, Patti. "Should You Exercise? For PWCs, It's an Important but Individual Question." *The CFIDS Chronicle* 11, no. 3 (May/June 1998).

Schoenberger, N., et al. "Flexyx Neurotherapy System in the Treatment of Traumatic Brain Injury: An Initial Evaluation." *Journal of Head Trauma Rehabilitation* 16, no. 3 (2001): 260–74.

Stonecypher, Sherron M. "Treatment of Fibromyalgia: Managing a Multifactorial." United Kingdom Department of Health. *A Report of the CFS/ME Working Group, Report to the Chief Medical Officer of an Independent Working Group.* January 2002.

U.S. Department of Health and Human Services. "CFS Treatment." Centers for Disease Control report, February 2002.

U.S. Department of Health and Human Services. "Recovery from CFS." Centers for Disease Control report, February 2002.

White, K.P., et al. "Trauma and Fibromyalgia: Is There an Association and What Does It Mean?" *Seminars in Arthritis and Rheumatism* 29, no. 4 (February 2000): 200–16.

Chapter 13

Dobbins, J. G, et al. "Physical, Behavioral, and Psychological Risk Factors for Chronic Fatigue Syndrome: A Central Role for Stress?" *Journal of Chronic Fatigue Syndrome* 1 (1995): 43–58.

Goode, Erica. "The Heavy Cost of Chronic Stress," *New York Times*, December 17, 2002, section F, page 1.

Gyatso, Tenzin (The Dalai Lama). "The Monk in the Lab," *New York Times,* April 26, 2003, section A, page 19.

Chapter 14

"1999 Chronicle Reader Survey." *The CFIDS Chronicle* 12, no. 4 (July/August 1999).

Davis, Scott E., Esq. "Chronic Fatigue Syndrome and Fibromyalgia Patients: Should You File a Disability Claim?" Immune*Support*.com. September 2002.

Davis, Scott. E., Esq. "Winning Your CFS Disability Case: Five Crucial Steps You Need to Know." *The CFIDS Chronicle* 13, no. 2 (Spring 2000).

"FMS/CFS Treatment Approaches." *Fibromyalgia Network*, October 1999.

Hall, Bob. "Fibromyalgia from a Man's Point of View." National Fibromyalgia Association Web site. Web site information. http://fmaware.org/patient/coping/fm_fromaman.htm

Hoh, David. "Treatment at the Cheney Clinic." *The CFIDS Chronicle* 11, no. 4 (July/August 1998).

Lapp, C. W. "Pregnancy and CFIDS." Transcript from the CFIDS information line, #9505. The CFIDS Association of America, 1994.

Masi, A. T., et al. "Person-Centered Approach to Care, Teaching, and Research in Fibromyalgia Syndrome: Justification from Biopsychosocial Perspectives in Populations." *Seminars on Arthritis and Rheumatism*, 32, no. 2 (October 2002): 71–93.

"Testimony of Honorable Robert T. Matsui of California, regarding the Attorney Fee Payment System Improvement Act 2001." *Congressional Record*, November 16, 2001.

"Testimony of Honorable E. Clay Shaw of Florida, regarding the Attorney Fee Payment System Improvement Act 2001." *Congressional Record*, November 16, 2001.

Underhill, Rosemary. "CFIDS and Pregnancy: Questions and concerns." *The CFIDS Chronicle* 11, no. 1 (January/February 1998).

Chapter 15

Allen, Jamie. "Author Escapes Illness with Stirring 'Seabiscuit.'" CNN.com, May 4, 2001.

Blumenthal, Amy. "Leading on the Backstretch: Laura Hillenbrand and Seabiscuit come home winners." *Kenyon College Alumni Bulletin* 22, no. 4 (Spring 2001).

Duenwald, Mary. "Power of Positive Thinking Extends, It Seems, to Aging." *New York Times*, November 19, 2002, science desk, section F, page 1.

Siegel, Bernie, M.D., "Conscious Healing." Ethoschannel.com, 2001.

Teitelbaum, Jacob, M.D. *Three Steps to Happiness! Healing Through Joy.* Annapolis, MD: Deva Press, 2003.

Chapter 16

Allen, Jamie. "Author Escapes Illness with Stirring 'Seabiscuit.'" CNN.com, May 4, 2001.

Bell, David S., M.D., et. al. "Thirteen-Year Follow-up of Children and Adolescents with Chronic Fatigue Syndrome." *Pediatrics* 107, no. 5, (May 2001): 994–998.

"CFS: a Real Disease." Videotape produced by The CFS Foundation, Inc., 10 Wild Partridge Ct., Greensboro, NC 27455, (800) 597-4CFS, 1992.

"Chronic Fatigue Syndrome: Diagnosing the Doubt." CTV World Television, A Health News Production, USC Instructional Television Network, Los Angeles, 1991.

Cohen, Kenneth S. "Qigong for CFIDS: Ancient Wisdom Meets Modern Science." *The CFIDS Chronicle* 11, no. 5 (September/October 1998).

Collinge, William. "Take Heart: Recovery from Chronic Fatigue Syndrome Happens." Immune*Support*.com, September 20, 2002.

Duenwald, Mary. "Power of Positive Thinking Extends, It Seems, to Aging." *New York Times*, November 19, 2002, science desk, section F, page 1.

Fennell, Patricia A. "CFS Sociocultural Influences and Trauma: Clinical Considerations." *Journal of Chronic Fatigue Syndrome* 1, no. 3/4 (April 1995).

Fox, Betty Sue. "Living with CFIDS: Writing as Self-help for Persons with CFIDS." *The CFIDS Chronicle* 12, no. 5 (September/October 1999).

Hoh, David. "Effective treatment: Unusual Controlled Study Tests Entire Protocol." *The CFIDS Chronicle* 11, no. 5 (September/October 1998).

Masuda, A., et al. "The Prognosis After Multidisciplinary Treatment for Patients with Postinfectious Chronic Fatigue Syndrome and Noninfectious Chronic Fatigue Syndrome." *Journal of Behavioral Medicine* 25, no. 5 (October 2002): 487–97.

"Pro Health's HEALTHwatch Treatment Guide." Immune*support*.com http://www.immunesupport.com/healthwatch, 2002.

Reyes, M. et al. "Chronic Fatigue Syndrome Progression and Self-Defined Recovery: Evidence from the CDC Surveillance System." *Journal of Chronic Fatigue Syndrome* 5 (1999): 17–27.

Teitelbaum, J., et al. "Effective Treatment of Chronic Fatigue Syndrome (CFIDS) & Fibromyalgia (FMS)—A Randomized, Double-Blind, Placebo-Controlled, Intent to Treat Study," *Journal of Chronic Fatigue Syndrome* 8, no. 2 (2001).

Wood, B., et al. "Personality and Social Attitudes in Chronic Fatigue Syndrome." *Journal of Psychosomatic Research* 47 (1999): 385–87.

INDEX